Invisible
No
More

Invisible No More

EMBRACING YOUR ROAD *to* RECOVERY *from* LONG COVID *and* OTHER COMPLEX CHRONIC ILLNESSES

Ilene Sue Ruhoy, MD, PhD

ST. MARTIN'S
ESSENTIALS
NEW YORK

First published in the United States by St. Martin's Essentials, an imprint of St. Martin's Publishing Group

INVISIBLE NO MORE. Copyright © 2025 by Ilene Sue Ruhoy. All rights reserved. Printed in the United States of America. For information, address St. Martin's Publishing Group, 120 Broadway, New York, NY 10271.

www.stmartins.com

The Library of Congress Cataloging-in-Publication Data is available upon request.

ISBN 978-1-250-91091-2 (hardcover)
ISBN 978-1-250-91092-9 (ebook)

Our books may be purchased in bulk for promotional, educational, or business use. Please contact your local bookseller or the Macmillan Corporate and Premium Sales Department at 1-800-221-7945, extension 5442, or by email at MacmillanSpecialMarkets@macmillan.com.

First Edition: 2025

10 9 8 7 6 5 4 3 2 1

Writing this book was both cathartic and therapeutic for me and allowed me to feel deeply grateful for those who have been a part of my journey. I easily cry at the support and hand-holding from my husband, Steven, and my daughter, Madeline, both of whom have made this life worth living in ways I could not possibly have fathomed as a younger person growing up on the streets of Brooklyn, New York. They are the reasons I take each breath and each step. I would absolutely not be who I am today if I had not met Steven and had not had Madeline. I honestly don't know how I got so lucky.

And truth be told, I am at this point in my career because of my patients. Their trust in me, their belief in me, their willingness to share their stories with me and allow me into their lives and to witness their suffering has given me the greatest gifts—a journey into humanity as it should be seen and should be acknowledged.

Contents

Introduction

SOPHIE ARRIVED IN MY CLINIC one day in a state of despair. Her complexion was pale, and her eyes were heavy and red as she dropped into the chair across from me. "So," I started, "what brings you here to see me?"

Instead of answering, she burst into tears. She pulled a tissue from her purse and dabbed her eyes, and when she calmed down she told me that she felt lost and scared. Despite vaccination, she had contracted Covid—a mild case, she recalled. "It felt like a bad flu that lasted two, maybe three days," she said. Her recovery was slow but steady. She experienced some fatigue over the next couple of weeks, but soon she felt confident that she had returned to her baseline. And then, about two months later, something scary happened. She was at the university library where she worked when she was overcome with sudden dizziness and had to sit down. She felt confused, she couldn't remember what she'd been doing just then, and her heart was racing. Fearful she was having a stroke or a heart attack, she went to the local ER. Her evaluation was normal; she was told it was anxiety, and she was discharged home.

Over the following weeks and months, Sophie continued to experience episodes of increased heart rate, flushing, headache, dizziness, and confusion, and soon the symptoms had increased in severity to the point that she was barely able to get herself out of bed in the morning or stand in the kitchen long enough to make breakfast for her young son. It seemed like everything she ate made her nauseated. She developed shortness of breath, but when she went to the clinic or to urgent care, her oxygen always read as normal. By the time she came to me she had seen several doctors, but, because her labs and testing were consistently normal, all of them had told her that her problem was simply the stress of being a young working mom.

"This isn't any kind of stress I've ever felt," she insisted to me. "At this point, I don't know what to do. I feel like my life is no longer my own."

Regardless of what those doctors had told her, Sophie knew there was something wrong, and it wasn't stress. It was Long Covid, and even though I, along with everybody else at that time, knew almost nothing about that new condition, I was still able to offer her the thing she needed most: I believed her. As an integrative medicine specialist, environmental toxicologist, and neurologist trained in both pediatric and adult neurological and mitochondrial disease, I had been working with patients with chronic and complex disease for decades and had become, somewhat unwittingly and unintentionally, an expert in what some think of as "mysterious diseases" and what many— even highly experienced doctors—think of as symptoms based in fear, anxiety, and stress. These diseases may indeed be mysterious, but they are real. As real as they get, especially to the individuals who suffer and those who love them.

Post-Exposure Illness

MANY "MYSTERIOUS" DISEASES ARE DISTINCTLY post-viral, occurring after colds or flus or a stomach bug, for example, and exist under a broader umbrella of what I call "post-exposure illnesses." Many patients come to me with stories of contracting a gastrointestinal issue while traveling abroad and their digestion never being the same, or of a fever they had in grad school that seemed to fundamentally alter their ability to concentrate for the rest of their career. They have a clear sense that it was after that specific infectious illness, but when I take a comprehensive history there is usually evidence of multiple exposures—both infectious and environmental. Their suffering is compounded when their healthcare providers are unable to understand their symptoms or, worse, seem to minimize or doubt them.

Maybe something like this has happened to you. Maybe you had strep throat or a sinus infection, or you had Covid, and then you got better. And then, some time later, you felt . . . not right. Your symptoms may have been obscure or vague at first—fatigue, a nagging brain fog, difficulty focusing and staying on task, frequent headaches—but they persisted despite your best attempts at taking care of yourself, and soon they worsened. So you made an appointment with a doctor and arrived filled with hope that this doctor would be able to help you. Instead, after discussing your concerns with you, the doctor said, "You're fine. There's nothing wrong with you." Maybe they added, not so helpfully, "You need to exercise more. Reduce your stress and anxiety." Maybe you even pushed back gently. You requested certain tests, and the doctor acquiesced, but the tests came back normal. "I told you," your doctor may have said. "All looks well." They may even have referred you to a psychiatrist, as if it were all in your head.

It's infuriating.

And yet, these experiences are becoming more common. Chronic symptoms combined with this kind of healthcare experience have left many patients feeling alone and hopeless. If this sounds familiar, I want to acknowledge that loneliness, because I know how dark that pit can be. I feel for you. But let me also assure you that you are far from alone. In addition to the countless patients I have seen, heard, and helped, and the millions of people who have developed Long Covid (about 7 percent of U.S. adults, according to a 2022 survey[1]), something similar happened to me. I spent more than a year telling colleagues that I was not feeling well, and I was repeatedly told it was stress, or it was anxiety, or it was perimenopause. It was not. It was a seven-centimeter brain tumor that required urgent surgery, radiation, and then more radiation. I went through post-operative pain that was undertreated and so severe that I would have done anything to end it—including ending my life if I had been physically able. That pain clouded my love and devotion for my family and my life. If just one doctor had listened to me sooner, I could have avoided much of that.

So, no, you are not alone, and more important, your situation is not hopeless. When I finally recovered from my surgery and returned to work in my clinic, I began seeing more and more patients with chronic complex illness. With some digging, I realized that most of these patients had had some kind of exposure in the past, had recovered, but then fell into a life with symptoms that seemed disconnected from any specific illness or cause. I mentioned fatigue, brain fog, and headaches. Other symptoms include physical weakness, rashes, light sensitivity, shortness of breath, ringing in the ears, tremor, palpitations, body and joint pain, post-exertional malaise, cough, dizziness, stomach pain, constipation, change in menstrual cycle, and more.

---

1 "Long Covid in Adults: United States, 2022," Centers for Disease Control and Prevention, September 2023.

Among those early patients was a string of complex illness patients with symptoms that met criteria for a diagnosis of myalgic encephalomyelitis/chronic fatigue syndrome (ME/CFS). It didn't take long to notice that these patients shared a common thread. They were mostly highly functional people with robust lives and great potential, and then they got sick. It was often mononucleosis, recurrent streptococcal infections, Lyme or other tick-borne infection, or sometimes a severe gastrointestinal infection while traveling. Sometimes it was a different exposure such as mold or another contaminant or toxicant. Regardless, there was an exposure at some point in the patient's life, and they went on to develop myriad chronic symptoms that completely changed the course of their health. These patients rarely found reassurance and care and often worsened as they sought treatment, first from the conventional medical establishment and then, after confronting the lack of understanding and curiosity from their medical doctors, from alternative healthcare providers, all with the great hope that someone would take an interest in trying to improve their quality of life.

By working deliberately with these patients and the myriad others who have come to me with post-exposure illness—by listening to them and sticking with them through wrong turns and following up on small successes—I have been able to help most of them begin to recover, and in the process, I developed a reputation for treating patients with these tricky illnesses. I have also developed a broad collection of strategies that work, though it commonly takes trial and error with an individual patient to find what works for them.

Integrative Neurologist

I AM OFTEN REFERRED TO as an "integrative neurologist." I think it is mainly due to my additional training in integrative medicine with Dr. Andrew Weil at the University of Arizona, but I also like to think it is because I very much enjoy the challenge of thinking outside my "box" or my "silo." I like to incorporate other treatment options and management techniques beyond pharmaceuticals. I further trained in medical acupuncture, herbal formulations, and mind–body connection to do just that, but to be sure I did it responsibly and with practical know-how.

My integrative bent was also very much fostered by my dissertation work while completing my PhD in environmental toxicology. I had chosen this topic because I was an amateur environmentalist for most of my life and wanted to learn more. I had already earned my MD when I entered this PhD program, and by that time I was fully convinced that our environment contributes to what makes us sick: the air we breathe, the water we drink, the soil in which our food is grown, what could grow in our abodes, and the way in which we treat animals for the presumed need of animal protein. My dissertation work was on pharmaceutical residues in our waters, of which there are way more than you would expect. I also had the great fortune of working with the Environmental Protection Agency (EPA) and some of the best environmental scientists in the country. I learned a great deal about how our environment has changed over the decades, how it has gotten dirtier and continues to worsen, especially with budgetary constraints on the EPA. I knew I wanted to combine all my training to help public health, even if it was initially one patient at a time. Today I bring my neurology expertise, my environmental toxicology expertise, and my additional training in integrative and alternative modalities to each patient appointment.

Given my integrative focus and my desire to learn as much as I can about what makes us sick, perhaps it was inevitable that I came to specialize in patients with complex, "mysterious" illnesses. I feel compelled to help those patients. And I feel compelled to solve these puzzles.

A New Enlightenment

MEDICINE HAS HISTORICALLY FOCUSED ONLY on acute illness from an infection. Post-infectious symptoms have almost systematically been ignored, and there has been a collective eye roll when individuals say they still feel lousy once the evidence of an active infection subsides—that is, the rash is gone, the fever is resolved, the blood and urine are clear. The symptoms patients present with post-infection create uncertainty for doctors, and, honestly, their very identity as a doctor who treats diseases can feel threatened. Compound this with the stress of practicing medicine today, with the insurance obstacles, hospital administration demands, and documentation requirements, and most doctors do not have the bandwidth or the motivation to take the time to investigate, learn more, understand more, listen more, and just help more.

But that is not to say we don't know that post-viral complications happen. For example, over the decades we have collected data showing that Guillain-Barré syndrome (GBS), a type of peripheral neuropathy, often seems to happen after a gastrointestinal infection. This has been so apparent that it is an oft-seen board examination question for neurologists. Patients are always asked if they have a history of GBS before they get a flu shot, and that is because we know there are reports of this acute neuropathy disease following vaccination.[2] For another example, when a child is admitted because they are unable to move a limb, and we see evidence of a lesion affecting the myelin surrounding neurons on their brain or spine, we ask if they have had a recent viral illness or a recent vaccination. That's because tests have found that demyelinating lesions are a distinct possibility following certain viruses due to "molecular mimicry," when a virus looks so much like another

2 Olajide Bamidele Ogunjimi et al., "Guillain-Barré Syndrome Induced by Vaccination Against Covid-19: A Systematic Review and Meta-Analysis," *Cureus* 15, no. 4 (April 2023): https://www.ncbi.nlm.nih.gov/pmc/articles /PMC10183219/.

cell or component of your body that your immune system becomes confused and attacks those other cells even after the correct target (the bug) has been subdued.

These are diseases we see in the fairly short-term post-infectious period—they do not necessarily show up months or years later. But recent research, largely buoyed by Covid-19, has looked at the risk of delayed effects that may not be as acutely threatening as the initial infection but are no less threatening to quality—and, potentially, quantity—of life. There has been an explosion of support-ive data for the possible consequences of remote, delayed infection, most recently in January of 2022 and replicated since, when researchers finally declared that multiple sclerosis (MS) may be caused by the Epstein-Barr virus (EBV), for example.[3]

What is encouraging about this new "Enlightenment" era of multisystem medicine and science is that many sci-entists and physicians are no longer burying their heads in the sand or sitting within their self-constructed boxes, turning a blind eye to the reality of post-exposure ill-nesses. In many hospitals, diagnoses are no longer being avoided or negated, and there is more support than ever

---

3 Brian Doctrow, "Study Suggests Epstein-Barr Virus May Cause Mul-tiple Sclerosis," National Institutes of Health, February 1, 2022, https://www.nih.gov/news-events/nih-research-matters/study-suggests-epstein-barr-virus-may-cause-multiple-sclerosis; "Further Investigating the Link Between MS and Epstein-Barr," Harvard T. H. Chan School of Public Health, March 27, 2024, https://www.hsph.harvard.edu/news/hsph-in-the-news/further-investigating-the-link-between-ms-and-epstein-barr/.

before. We are learning so much, and at such a fast pace, that we will soon know enough to better treat and guide individuals who suffer with all manner of previously un-diagnosable "complicated" diseases showing as fatigue and other symptoms that may often get labeled as stress or anxiety or depression, or even psychosomatic illness. One of the unfortunate downsides of electronic medical records (EMRs) is that once a diagnosis of, for example, anxiety is on a patient's chart, it stays there in perpetuity, and over the years doctors may interpret all symptoms as related to that diagnosis.

Strategies That Work

UNTIL THEN, OF COURSE, PATIENTS like you are not satisfied, and they have no reason to be. I am sure you have suffered from symptoms that you don't understand and that may interfere with your daily life and provoke all kinds of emotions, including fear, anxiety, depression, and even irritation. You may first turn to Google, as we tend to do, but Google usually presents us with the best-case scenario or the worst-case scenario of any health-related thing you type into the search bar. The truth is that the vast major-ity of what is happening to your body lies somewhere in between. Nuance, as we know, is not favored by internet algorithms, whereas each of us is truly an individual. Even treating something as mundane as headaches requires an individual history: When do they happen? What happens right before and right after? How exactly do they feel? What makes it better or worse? How do you sleep? How do you eat, move, and manage stress? What is your family history, what is your medical history, what exposures have you had? And so on. The history for you will never be the exact same as the history for someone else. And because we are all individuals, the way a virus or other exposure affects us initially, and whether and how it affects us in subsequent assaults, can differ vastly.

That is why we need our doctors to look us in the eye and listen when we say something is not right. After all, you are the only person who inhabits your body, and just like Sophie, you know when something is not right. You may need someone to help you figure out how to fix it, but you are the authority on you.

Medicine has come so far in many ways, yet we remain so ill-informed, ill-advised, and led astray. I believe the gap between patient and doctor has widened to a point where our conversations are lost in translation, and that does not help either side. Patients hope to learn from their physicians, and physicians should embrace the idea that there is much to learn from patients. My hope is that *Invisible No More* will inspire both patients and doctors to help each other.

All of which sounds great to you, I'm sure, but in the meantime, you can't wait for some sunshiny future in which healthcare is not broken. Listen, life is short. That's more than just a phrase on a T-shirt, as I have learned acutely. While I have been writing this book, my younger sister passed away, and I have been referred to palliative care. So here: I wrote this book to help you take charge of your own health and recovery. It is full of practical, hands-on strategies both large and small that you can use to treat your illness. It also features strategies for talking to healthcare providers in order to get more personal, diligent care from them. There is much that you can do on your own to start feeling better today, and feel better again the day after that, and continue to feel better. This book is a compilation of what I have seen in my practice, what I believe to be true or sound, and what I recommend to my patients. It's a compilation of things that work.

I know you are hungry for healing and desperate for answers, and that's what I am offering. This book is not a road map to recovery, because there is no road map. Remember, we're all individuals with unique genetics and unique lifetimes of exposures. There may be no road map, but you can make it to your destination anyway. You do it one step at a time. And that's what this book is: a collection of steps, all of which have been proven to help patients, including myself, get better.

Maybe your symptoms are mild but persistent, or maybe you're on the other end of the spectrum: You're bedbound. You live with the shades drawn and dwindling hope of ever feeling better. Maybe you have Long Covid or chronic fatigue syndrome. Maybe you have mast cell activation disorder, or maybe you don't know what you have. I'm telling you, however you are doing, it is within you to make progress toward recovery, even if you're beaten down, exhausted, and miserable right now. There are strategies in this book that will work for you. They may not be easy. No pill, no surgery, no miracle cure is going to do it all. It takes hard work, tenacity, maybe some hard choices. It may mean making yourself uncomfortable in the short term in order to finally feel more comfortable. The good news is, it's up to you. And I know you can do it.

PART I

Something Is Not Right

1

The Neurologist
Becomes the Patient

MANY OF THE PATIENTS WHO come to see me in my practice today are on their fourth or fifth healthcare professional in their quest to figure out what the hell is wrong with them. They've seen a general practitioner, and they've seen various specialists and nurses and techs. All that *seeing*, yet they've rarely felt seen. When a patient's symptoms are mysterious and vague and don't add up to an easily diagnosable illness with a plug-and-play treatment, doctors often give up. They send you to another specialist. Or worse, tell you it's all in your head. By the time they get to me, my patients have endured tests and exams and countless questions, yet they're no closer to an answer. More important, they're no closer to relief. It's not in their head. They are frustrated and often angry. They feel defeated. Sometimes they cry or tremble in my office as they recount what they've been through, their hands gripping the chair arms. They look at me with dark, exhausted eyes. And I look back. I try to see them and help them feel seen, to listen and help them feel heard.

This is my life's mission.

Part of why I feel so passionate about this may be because when I was a child, I rarely felt seen. My family was beyond dysfunctional, and I didn't feel safe at home. I did not know where I belonged, and I did not know where I was wanted. I always felt out of place, the odd one. I never wanted a birthday party, because I was sure no one would show up. And my mother never tried to convince me otherwise. My father was an alcoholic, a gambler, a liar, and a womanizer. He cheated repeatedly on my mother, and I'll never forget the day I watched him pack his things to move out of our apartment after one last fight with her. The sleeves of his blue oxford were rolled to the elbows, and his forearms were pale and hairy but strong. "All men need an alternative life to their married one," he said to me. I was five.

My mother had immigrated to the United States from Israel at age sixteen. Her parents were Holocaust survivors; this fact created a weight that she carried, and she felt unworthy. Her parents were forever changed by the trauma they experienced in the camps, and it affected the way they parented, as they alternated between being fearful of the world and being militant in their efforts to change it. This left her feeling unsafe in a place where she had every reason to feel safe. A beautiful young woman with large green eyes, blond hair, and a slim build, she was still in high school and barely spoke English when my father proposed to her, and she accepted. He convinced her she was lucky he found her. Throughout my life, she has had low self-esteem that was made better only by having a man in her life. She did not, and still does not, ever want to be alone. After my father left, she dated often, and eventually a man moved into our apartment. He was a New York City police officer with a temper, and let's just say it was not a relaxed and peaceful home for my formative years. When he left her, she soon met another man, married him, and moved to another borough, taking my younger sister. I was in high school by this time and had to move in with my father if I didn't want to leave the one place I felt I belonged: the school where I'd grown to admire many of my teachers, who were my mentors and my inspiration to persist and be present in my life.

School was my escape from the life I led at home. I immersed myself in books because they allowed me to be someone else, somewhere else. When my teachers suggested that I go to college, I was surprised. No one in my family had ever gone to college. No one even talked about college, so it wasn't something I had ever thought of. But I went because my teachers told me I should, and a few good friends were going, and I'm glad I did, because the promises of the world opened up to me.

After graduating college, I applied to medical school

because I wanted to make an impact in the lives of others, but also because I was oddly curious about other lives. I didn't know if my life was unusual or not that unusual, and I wanted to find out. I also knew that I needed to forge my own path. I wanted my value to be held in who I was and what I stood for. I interviewed at the University of Pittsburgh School of Medicine in the dead of winter. It was sixteen degrees and I was freezing, but there was something about the city and its people that drew me in. That, and the fact that it was not New York, sealed the deal.

In my second year as a medical student, I met my husband, a pathology resident; he has been my rock and my unwavering supporter ever since. And eventually I became a doctor. If someone had told my twelve-year-old self, living in our chaotic apartment with my younger sister, my mother, and my mother's unpredictable boyfriend, that someday I would persevere and make a life for myself, I would not have believed it.

But I did persevere, just as I did years later when I became sick. That's why I'm still here. I don't think all of life happens because of conscious, intentional choices. I just take one day at a time, see what the day's challenge is, and try to meet it head-on the best I can. I don't think that makes me special, by the way. I see that resilience and fortitude in my patients every day. Their strength only adds to mine. It's what keeps me going.

A few years before my grandparents died, I interviewed them about their experience at Auschwitz. "How did you do it?" I asked. "How did you go on for another day?" Their answer was simple. They each said it was because they had no choice, and because they had hopes for a brighter future and a higher purpose. And that purpose, they said, was me.

I'm here now to pay it forward.

Searching for Answers

I LEARNED EARLY ON THAT I very much enjoy thinking outside the box as a neurologist, but practicing conventional neurology at the university clinic did not leave much room for me to go beyond the expected standard of care for this symptom or that diagnosis. More importantly to me, I did not see patients getting better. It is often stated in neurology that we have a lot of diagnoses but not a whole lot of treatments. That was hard for me to accept, so I began pursuing knowledge about other methods of treatment by taking classes in integrative medicine and eventually doing an integrative medicine fellowship with Dr. Andrew Weil at the University of Arizona. I gained a whole new education on diseases I did not really understand or even know about before. Some of these diagnoses were intentionally disregarded in the conventional world, and patients who claimed they suffered with one of them were sometimes met with ridicule.

One example of this is the controversial diagnosis pediatric acute-onset neuropsychiatric syndrome (PANS), which occurs after streptococcal and other infections. I saw patients with symptoms that matched this diagnosis when I was working at a children's hospital (I trained in both pediatric and adult neurology). These children would have tics, erratic behavior, tremendous anxiety, poor sleep, inattentiveness, restrictive dietary choices, and sometimes violent outbursts. One boy sat in my office chewing his cheek compulsively, unable to stop even when his mother specifically reminded him. He had not slept more than a few hours a night in weeks, and his equally exhausted mother told me that he had developed motor tics and severe anxiety to the point he was unable to leave the house or go to school or play soccer, which he used to love to do. The boy stared at the floor, his mouth riddled with sores from his chewing. "His doctor told me it was a behavioral issue," the mother said desperately. "He made me feel like this is all due to bad parenting."

This diagnosis from pediatricians, I learned, was typical. At that time, many doctors and institutions would not even see patients if the reported concern was PANS. Many of the kids were referred to psychiatry. But when I saw these patients in the clinic and listened to their parents describe what was going on, I started to notice a similar thread to their stories. These kids were essentially neurotypical and high functioning, both socially and academically, and then at some point they developed an infectious illness—strep throat or another upper respiratory illness—and soon after that they woke up a different child. Normal, then sick, then not normal. I heard it time and time again, and there was no way, I thought, that it was a coincidence. Were these families meeting in a room somewhere and comparing notes about what they would tell their doctors? More to the point, the children were clearly in distress. They did not want to feel this way or act this way. They did not want to be taken to doctor after doctor while struggling at school and losing all of their friends. And for sure their parents did not want this to be happening to their children. The stress on the family was palpable. I could find no reason not to believe them, validate them, and help search for answers.

To expand my knowledge and ability to find those an-swers, I went on to get a PhD in environmental toxi-cology. I further trained in medical acupuncture, herbal formulations, and mind–body connection, and today I bring all these nodes of expertise to the table when seeing patients—neurology, environmental toxicology, and inte-grative and alternative treatments.

It Happens to Me

BY THE SPRING OF 2014, I had been a physician for ten years. Then one day at work, I realized that I felt different. I was between patients with a moment to myself when it hit me. I had this feeling of dragging fatigue that was not sleepiness, and not exhaustion. I could not put my finger on it, but something was not right, and I realized it had been like this for some time, slowly building. My thinking was cloudy; my motivation was drooping. The idea of getting up from my desk and walking to the bathroom felt like a huge chore. I was not weak, exactly, but I felt as if I could not do the next task.

As physicians do, I ignored these feelings as best I could and struggled to complete my days. And the days added up. There were moments when I was with patients when I knew I wasn't giving them my best, because I wasn't at my best. Sometimes I was inside my own head doing everything I could not to pass out, vomit, or cry. In between patients I would sit still with the lights out and try to relax, maybe do breathing exercises. Sometimes I went outdoors to get fresh air.

On days when the symptoms were not so debilitating, I tried to minimize what was happening by thinking maybe it was something I ate or how I had slept the night before. Maybe it was my level of stress, or maybe I was just getting older. The symptoms were similar to those of depression, but I knew I was not depressed. I was not sad. I looked forward to my days at work because helping patients truly felt rewarding to me. My home life was great, with an incredible partner in my husband and my beautiful ten-year-old daughter, who was happy and doing well, which is all a parent can ask for.

It was not depression, but it was *something*. I'd been healthy, fit, and highly productive my whole life, and I never really knew what being unwell felt like. I'd always had the privilege of good health, but I'd never truly appreciated it until now.

Over the ensuing weeks, this feeling of fatigue and unwellness came in spurts, usually unexpectedly and with no clear trigger. I started to keep a journal in the hope I would see a trend in my stress, diet, or sleep, but to no avail. I couldn't find a cause, and I couldn't find anything that would relieve my symptoms. As an integrative neurologist, I had a lot of ideas, and I was trying everything from restricting my diet to meditation to herbal remedies, even though I knew instinctively that none of these approaches was going to magically cure me. I was just trying to get enough relief to get through my days. Instead, things got worse. I couldn't sleep well at night. I developed temperature dysregulation, whereby I was cold when I should not be cold and hot when I should not be hot, and I couldn't run when the sun was out. I became very sensitive to light. I started getting migraine headaches preceded by a visual aura that left me totally unable to work. I came to expect that every day I would experience dizziness and nausea in the afternoon so severe that it forced me to find an empty room at the hospital and lie down in the dark. At the time, I was six months into a neuromuscular fellowship that I was really excited about, but I had to drop out. I needed to reduce my workload. I was starting to get scared.

So scared that I finally sought help. I assumed it would be easy for me to find help—I was a neurologist working in a hospital. Easy, right? I talked to a few colleagues about what was going on, but they all suggested that I was stressed out because of the demands of work. To be fair, I did not seek them out as a patient and was just "curbsiding," as we say in medicine when just asking a specialist about their opinion on something. Naturally, on some level I felt relieved that they did not think it was anything more serious than stress, but that only made me feel shame, because it suggested I was somehow less resilient than my colleagues. After all, we were all working the same hospital job.

One morning at home, my husband made me a toasted sesame bagel. It was a kind gesture and a food that I love, and I was looking forward to the breakfast. When he slid the plate to me, though, and I saw that it was slightly burned, something exploded inside me. He gave me a *burned bagel*? I had never felt so angry in all my life. "You burned it!" I screamed, and I threw it. The bagel bounced off his chest, a splatter of hummus left behind on his shirt. To his credit, he didn't respond with anger of his own. He barely reacted at all, other than to apologize. He knew that wasn't me.

In fact it was clear that I had changed. I was moody. I was impatient, irritable, condescending, and generally not fun to be around. In short, I was an asshole. I contained it for patients, but when I came home, the cup runneth over.

So I went to my primary doctor. Like my colleagues, he told me that it all had to do with stress and my lifestyle habits, including nutrition and exercise. He gave me a bunch of lifestyle recommendations, all of which I knew and most of which I'd tried. But, in my effort to be a good patient, I did my best to improve what was already a decent diet, added more meditation, and incorporated more yoga and walking. Yet my symptoms continued to progress. I went back to my primary care doctor, and he ran labs, which were all normal, and he sheepishly recommended I see a neurologist.

I visited a neurologist whom I knew as a colleague but not personally. Trim and fit, he stared into his computer screen while I talked, drumming the fingers of one hand on the desk while mousing with the other. I tried to be unemotional and rational as I explained what I had been experiencing and how my symptoms were getting worse and more frequent. When I was finished he said, while still looking at the computer screen instead of me, "You're overthinking these symptoms. As a neurologist, you know too much." He also referred to my history of migraines. He went on to say something about textbooks, but I was so stunned at the way he was writing me off that I was barely listening. Regaining my wits, I respectfully countered that my history of migraines was maybe one or two per year, but now I was experiencing atypical head pain and neurological symptoms weekly. His response to this was "Well, you are getting older." I am a woman, and hormones change, this is true. But it was clear he wasn't listening to me. I knew this was more than hormones. He suggested working less and exercising more, and starting migraine medication.

At this point, I realized he was ending the meeting without even giving me a neurological exam, which is standard when seeing someone for neurological issues.

I was shocked. I said, "Don't you even want to examine me?"

"Well, I figured since you're a neurologist you would tell me if there's a problem," he said.

At my urging, he conducted a very basic exam by testing my reflexes and strength, but he didn't look into the back of my eyes, which is the only part of the exam that I can't do to myself. And then he told me to come back if my symptoms did not improve.

They did not improve, but I did continue to work, travel, and socialize. Simply put, my life called for it. One day I had lunch with a close friend. After we finished and hugged goodbye, I turned to leave the table and suddenly tripped and fell to the floor. There was nothing there; I hadn't tripped over anything. It was as if my foot just decided not to work. I was embarrassed, and my friend rushed to my aid. I assured her I was okay, brushed myself off, and continued to walk down the street. I was feeling very dizzy, and a sense of panic and fear came over me.

The next doctor I saw was an ear, nose, and throat (ENT) specialist. Sometimes headaches can be caused by sinus inflammation, and even though I did not have a history of sinus issues, I figured it was worth a try. But it wasn't. Like the neurologist, he told me I was reading too much into my symptoms. He did a basic ENT exam and ordered a sinus scan. I asked for an MRI, but he insisted all I needed was the sinus scan. The sinus scan showed a little fluid in one of my sinus cavities behind my cheek. He diagnosed a sinus infection and put me on fluoroquino-lone, an antibiotic about which there were well-known and oft-reported concerns regarding toxicity.

"That doesn't make sense," I said. I didn't have the symptoms of a sinus infection. I asked if the findings on the sinus scan could be related to possible inflammation in my brain, and he told me I was being dramatic and "a little hysterical." My pulse quickened at that extremely offensive comment, but I clenched my fist and remained calm—the very model of a nonhysterical woman.

"Take the antibiotic," he said.

In my desperation, I started the medication, but by day three I began to experience fevers, dizziness, and nausea. I called the ENT's nursing line, and the nurse told me that these symptoms could not be from the antibiotic despite the clear timing of their onset with when I take the pills. In a definitive and dismissive manner, she said it was not a typical side effect of this antibiotic. However, since I was a physician, she said I could elect to continue the medication or not. It was interesting to me to note that my status as a physician held value when it served those who were supposed to treat me. When they did not want to make a definitive decision or did not want to consider and discuss what could be happening, then it was up to me. But when I asked for particular diagnostic orders, then I should leave the medicine up to them and I should just behave as the patient.

I elected to stop the medication, and the symptoms did

indeed improve. But I was back to my original symptoms and fears. I became hopeless and depressed and even more irritable with my husband. I went back to my primary care provider and asked him to order an MRI, but he did not think it was indicated and seemed to rely on the specialists I had seen to make that determination.

A Doctor Who Listens!

BY THIS TIME I HAD asked several doctors for an MRI, but none had ordered one. One doctor even told me, "I'm not going to feed into your hysteria by ordering an MRI." Imagine saying that to a neurologist! And yet, I continued to stubbornly trust in the professionals of my own chosen profession. Looking back, it's easy to say I should have pushed harder. Why didn't I? They were telling me that it was not a big deal, and deep down I wanted to believe them.

That July I went away on a weekend to New Mexico for an intensive herbal formulations class for physicians who want training in non-pharmaceutical methods. It's a popular class, which I had signed up for back in January, and I was really looking forward to it. At this point in my career I was deep into learning about integrative medicine. I had completed that fellowship with Dr. Andrew Weil, and this intensive class with the well-known Dr. Tieraona Low Dog at her ranch in Santa Fe was an exciting opportunity.

I was having about ten migraines a month by this time, and they were horrible and debilitating. So in addition to the pain, I was also extremely disappointed when I had one in the morning before class that weekend. I didn't want to miss class. I took a bunch of Advil and lay in bed for a few hours, and ultimately I did make it to the course. But this was the day when things went from bad to worse, and I realized that something was deeply, deeply wrong.

We were standing in the sun on Dr. Low Dog's ranch, listening to her as she talked about the chamomile plant, when suddenly my hand, which was holding a book, seized up. *My muscles must be having a reaction to the heat,* I thought. My hand must be overworked from holding the book for so long. I know now that I was having a focal seizure, but at the time I just thought it was weird. Dr. Low Dog continued to explain the medicinal qualities of the plants we were standing among as I tried with my other hand to pry my fingers open. Finally I got the book out and shook and rubbed my hand. A few minutes later, the cramping released.

Later that evening, I drove to Whole Foods to get something to eat. I walked into the store, and suddenly it was filled with a very loud reverberating sound. It was so loud and penetrating that it physically hurt. I could feel the sound actually radiating down my throat into my heart. I thought it was coming from the speakers, and I looked around at the other shoppers to see if it was as painful for them as it was for me. I had a look on my face like, *Can you believe this store's speaker system?* But everyone seemed to be completely unbothered by this very loud, reverberating sound. They weren't reacting at all. I couldn't make sense of it. Finally the noise stopped, and I quickly finished my shopping. By the time I left the store I was reeling with nausea, and I vomited in the parking lot. That's when I realized that the sound had been inside me. In that moment, I felt true terror.

Somehow I made it back to my hotel. As I drove there, I realized that I had driven many miles that weekend yet had never gotten a grasp on landmarks or directions. I'd frequently been lost. I'd felt disconnected and dissociated from who I was and where I was. I was even finding it hard to remember the names of my friends and family. Lying in my hotel bed that night, I felt alone. And I knew for sure that my doctors were all wrong.

When I got home I immediately saw another internist. This was another doctor whom I knew professionally but not personally. She got me in on short notice, and I came into her office tingling with dizziness, exhaustion, and anxiety. Would she listen to me? Would she have any answers? What if it was bad? She wore her white coat and stood tall with both confidence and compassion. I told her everything that had happened and everything I had felt. I broke down and cried, hard, ending my description of my experiences by begging her to please order me an MRI. And to my great relief, she did. "When a neurologist asks you to order a brain MRI," she said, "you order a brain MRI." I will forever be grateful for her compassion.

An MRI at Last

IN AUGUST 2015, I WENT in for an MRI of the brain. I had not slept the night before, so in addition to the huge anxiety I felt, I was even more exhausted than usual. I showed up an hour early and sat in the waiting room trying to keep myself distracted with social media and the requisite doctor's office copy of *Good Housekeeping*. I had not told anyone, not even my mother, and nobody except my husband knew where I was. They finally called me in and gave me directions about changing into the gown, taking off my wedding band, using the locker, and so on. But when I got into the dressing room, I could not recall any of it. I stared blankly for a few moments before figuring out enough to put on the gown and come out. By this time, I was trembling.

The tech was youthful and kind in purple scrubs, and though I can't remember anything she said to me, I do remember feeling calmer after talking with her. She handed me headphones and asked if I wanted any music during the scan. I asked for Simon & Garfunkel. Then she directed me to lie on the table, and she inserted an IV into my arm. I put on the headphones, and sure enough, Simon & Garfunkel was playing, and that calmed me down, too, and somehow I convinced myself that everything was going to be okay.

I had ordered countless MRIs in my life, but I had never had one, so I knew they were noisy, but I wasn't prepared for just how noisy it really was. The deep, rhythmic, guttural sounds overshadowed the lovely seventies folk songs on my headphones.

Finally I was slid out of the machine, and this time a different MRI tech came into the room with me. "The radiologist just called," he said. "He wants you to go directly to the ER."

I felt my gut crumple, and I had to catch my breath for a moment. I still had the IV in my arm. "Why?" I asked.

The tech said he didn't know. He only knew that the radiologist had called and asked him to tell me to go directly to the ER. He kept his face blank so as not to betray any emotion.

I said, "You do know that I am a neurologist, right? I know you know."

He said he couldn't tell me anything, and once again I began to tremble and cry. I went back to the locker to change, but my hands were shaking so much that I couldn't dress myself. Instead, I picked up my phone and called my husband. When I heard him pick up, I began crying even harder. "They want me in the ER," I finally managed to croak. He said he would meet me there.

I don't remember getting dressed or finding my way to the emergency room. When I arrived, my husband was already there. The staff there was expecting me and led us to a clinic room, where we waited for about twenty minutes. Twenty minutes is not an unreasonable amount of time. The ER doctor and radiologist had to confer and look over my case. I knew that, but still, that was a hard twenty minutes.

The ER doctor came in with a laptop that he wheeled in on a cart. The laptop was open to a slice, or frame, from my MRI, and I caught a quick glimpse of what appeared to be a very ominous brain cancer called a glioblastoma multiforme, which is usually a terminal diagnosis. This thing was ugly and large. I gasped and involuntarily fell to the floor in tears thinking of my now eleven-year-old daughter. My mind was racing—I probably had six months to two years to live—as I heard my husband asking for permission to review the scans. My husband worked as a physician in that same hospital, and he started to scroll through the slices. Shortly, I heard him say, "This is very well circumscribed."

Glioblastomas usually are not well circumscribed, meaning they are not usually round with defined borders. So I got myself up off the floor and looked at the scans with him and the ER physician. It appeared to be a meningioma, a tumor of the meninges, which are the linings of the brain. It had grown to a very large size—about seven centimeters—and there was significant swelling. In fact, the swelling had caused so much pressure that the left side of my brain was on the right side of my skull, and there was downward pressure on the left brain, which threatened to push parts of my brain into compartments where they do not belong. This is called herniation, and it is usually not compatible with life.

The neurosurgery team was immediately paged, and the nurse practitioner arrived in the room while we were still going over the slides. The nurse practitioner gave me a basic neurological exam, which was normal, and she commented that based on my scan she was amazed that she was unable to find any abnormality. She could not believe I had not had a seizure. In fact, she was shocked I was still standing and talking. "It's fortunate you had the MRI when you did," she said, and I could not help thinking of all the times I had asked for one. Then she looked in my eyes to do a funduscopic exam, an exam that looks at the back of the eye (which should be done by every neurologist), and noted swelling of the optic nerves. This explained the light sensitivity and other symptoms I had been experiencing and was also very consistent with the elevated pressure in my head from the swelling caused by the giant tumor. Lying there in the bed in the emergency room, staring at the huge, grapefruit-size tumor pushing into my brain and causing my brain to swell so much that it moved to a place in my skull it should not be, I was struck by the fact that no one had bothered to do the one physical exam test I could not do myself. Not a single doctor I had seen looked into my eyes during an exam, either literally or figuratively. The one thing no one had bothered to do was the one thing that would have demonstrated a positive, objective exam finding.

The neurosurgeon arrived, and I will never forget his kind face. His eyes were brown and filled with compassion. His complexion showed the hope of young surgeons, yet he had the wrinkles of a surgeon who had seen his fair share of tragic cases. He said this was very likely a meningioma, a type of tumor that is usually benign, though most probably a high-grade one because of the way it was behaving. Usually, low-grade meningiomas do not grow, at least not fast, and many patients are told to just wait and watch with regularly scheduled surveillance MRIs. That is indeed the conventional training in neurology. It is often said, "If you are going to have a brain tumor, then this is the type you want." I was soon going to prove that was not necessarily accurate. It was clear at that moment to everyone in the room that this was the reason I had been so ill for more than a year. And it was also clear, though unsaid, at least at that tense moment, that had this tumor been identified even six months earlier, it would have likely been a much smaller size and the surgery would have been much easier.

The neurosurgeon wanted to admit me right away. He wanted to schedule me for a cerebral angiogram first thing in the morning so, as he said, "We can find the vessel that's feeding this beast and cauterize it." Then I'd go into surgery the next day to remove that beast. Though I obviously understood the urgency, I insisted that I had to go home and speak with my daughter and that I would return the next day. There was a 30 percent chance that I could herniate on the operating table, and recovery was not guaranteed. The prognosis was not certain.

The surgeon agreed on my taking one night, but he said, "You have to come back in the morning."

And I thought, *Of course I will!*

Some Dark Nights

BEFORE WE WENT HOME, I called my mom to tell her what was happening, which was a very difficult conversation. She quickly became hysterical, and I found myself in the odd position of having to calm her down. She wanted to fly out to Seattle right away, but I persuaded her to hold off until after the surgery. After hanging up with me, she immediately called my sister, with whom I'd had a rocky relationship most of our lives, partly because we were separated after our parents divorced. She'd lived with our mom, and I'd lived with our dad. She also had some mental health issues that had clouded our relationship. But she called me right away to say she was there for me. She too wanted to come out right away, but I told her the same thing I told our mom, which was to hold off. One of the good things to come out of all this was that my relationship with her was repaired and deepened, and I remained very close with her until she died a few years later.

Mom also called my dad, apparently, but he never called me, which was very hurtful. I haven't spoken with him since.

My husband and I went home, and I sat down with my daughter and told her about what was going on and what was about to happen. She did not really understand, and she did not really want to talk about it, which I understood. I tried my best to give her the basics and not to scare her.

I could not sleep that night, of course, so I got up. I walked into the kitchen and found a spiral notebook and a pen and, sitting at the island counter by the light of the stained-glass lamp that hung above the island, I wrote her a long letter. I told her about all the things that I had hoped to be able to share with her and teach her throughout her life. I told her how to be the best person she could be and how to value each day and confront obstacles, embrace disappointment, and reach out to others. I told her about love and what real love was, because I had found real love with her father after trials of something less than real. I told her the right person will be there to support her, cheer her on, love her unconditionally, and that I only wanted true happiness and joy for her. I told her how special she is and how she should expect to be treated by others but at the same time try to understand the perspective of others. I told her that I wished that I could have been there through her life every step of the way. I told her that I was her biggest supporter and her biggest fan, and I loved her to the moon and back. I put that letter in an envelope and sealed it, and I gave it to my husband in the morning. I told him that if I didn't make it out of the hospital, I wanted him to give it to her.

The next morning, he drove me to the hospital. We rode in silence. We parked in silence. We checked in in silence. I undressed and put on my hospital gown and was told to go to the MRI suite. I explained I was not there for an MRI, that I was to have a cerebral angiogram.

The nurse gave me a puzzled look and left me on the gurney in the hallway to confirm. She returned shortly after and let me know I was correct and wheeled me to the angiogram suite.

On the angiogram table I was given fentanyl and mid-azolam (a benzodiazepine that is very sedating), which knocked me out into a twilight state: I was still awake enough to hear the technicians talking and laughing about their weekend plans, all while I was in horrible pain and wanted to cry. The disconnect between my pain and their jovial banter felt like a chasm that was representative of the disconnect I'd felt trying to get doctors to listen to me and to see me. Indeed, it's representative of medicine in general.

The artery feeding the tumor was identified and burned shut, and I was brought up to the neuro ICU floor. I had a horrible migraine, and in the room alone, I cried all night.

The next morning at five o'clock I was taken to the operating room, where medical staff were milling about preparing for my surgery. Everyone was kind and calm. My neurosurgeon held my hand and told me that all was going to be fine, and he was going to take care of it. The anesthesiologist put an oxygen mask on my face, ad-ministered drugs through my IV, and told me to count backward from one hundred. I got to ninety-three. The surgery was more than seven hours long. The tumor had to be scraped off my brain, and a portion of one of my venous sinuses had to be removed—all because the tumor had grown so large.

The next thing I remember is being yelled at in the recovery room. Two nurses were shaking my shoulders and screaming, "Ilene, where are you?" No matter how hard I tried, I could not recall the name of the hospital I was in; all that kept coming to mind was the hospital where I trained at, which I knew was incorrect. But they kept screaming. I finally told them to please give me a few minutes to orient myself and to stop screaming in my face and shaking me. I was still very much under the anesthesia.

I was eventually wheeled to my room, and it was here that I experienced the darkest night of my life. I was not given any pain medications, because there is a pervasive fear among physicians of treating pain with narcotics, and the hospital protocol was very stingy with post-operative pain treatment. But I was in pain. Tremendous pain. My cranium had been cut ear-to-ear, which included all the muscles necessary for basic functions. I could not talk or chew, and the pain left me so that I could not think straight. My skull was bolted to a metal brace. I was scared, suffering, and in disbelief about what had transpired in my last seventy-two hours. Who was I anymore? Would I ever be the same?

I wanted to die. I mean, I really wanted to die. This was not sadness as I had felt before. This was severe depression and suicidal ideation. If it were not for the fact that I was literally incapable of physically committing suicide at that time, I believe that I would have tried to end my life. I did not care about my husband, my daughter, or anything. I just knew my suffering and pain were so deep, so severe, and so traumatic that I just did not want to be there anymore. It was not just the pain, but the dissociation, and the real feeling that I would never find joy, love, and connection again in life. I refused all nursing visits. I told my husband to go home. I did not want him to see me like this. I did not want visitors. Not only was I depressed and in anguish, I was also very angry.

This darkness lasted for two long days. Finally, my husband spoke to the doctors and demanded that my pain be treated. I was given opiate medication that night, and the pain almost immediately responded. It's impossible to describe the relief I felt. It was as if the lights turned on, the fog cleared, I remembered who I was, and I was no longer stuck in a dark cavern hoping never to return. I could not touch it yet, but I saw the hope in the midst of the despair. That hope was everything to me. The nursing staff told my husband the next morning that I had turned a corner during the night. The note on my chart said, "Patient affect improved." That was one way to put it. With pain subsiding, so did my fear and anger. I became calm, and I was able to sleep. I allowed my family in the room. And I was able to transition to non-opiate pain relief within a few days. I was still unable to chew and eat because cut muscles can take a while to heal. A friend brought me freshly made juices, and they made all the difference in terms of getting nutrition because the mushy hospital food was inedible.

My hospital stay over the next few days only deepened the feeling of disconnect I'd experienced all along. When I asked attendants, these people who were caring for me, what medications they were injecting into my IV, they did not know. Though I was unable to chew, they served me solid foods that required chewing. I could not get up to use the restroom on my own, yet I had no one reliable to assist me in a consistent manner. I was not allowed to sleep, because they were required to do hourly neuro checks on me, which meant asking me to squeeze their fingers, move my toes, and tell them what year it was and who was the sitting president. It was not the kind of recovery you'd hope for after such major surgery, but I learned a lot. I learned what it's like to be a patient in our healthcare system.

Five days after surgery, I was discharged and went home to begin my long road to recovery. I was now a resident in the strange world of cancer patients, a world characterized by the dichotomy of hope and despair. We are given treatments, from surgery to chemotherapy to radiation, from immunotherapy to clinical trials, that help us, to varying degrees, look forward to a healthier future. But the C-word is a scary one, and it hangs darkly over everything. At my follow-up appointments with my neuro-oncologist, I sat in the waiting room with thirty other oncology patients and their loved ones and looked around at their faces. Those who were accompanied by someone tended to wear some of that hope in their expressions, while those who were alone showed their sadness, their fear, their defeat, and their sense of isolation plainly. I could sense their desire to be cared for and, perhaps because I recognized it from my own experience, their desire to be seen and heard. Having people who love you as part of your journey is critical to support the hope and optimism for a chance at recovery.

To be sick is an isolating experience like no other. We are constantly counseled to find a social network, spend time with our families, build community, and be grateful. But when we are sick—especially chronically sick—those bonds are less tight and less tangible. It is harder to find joy in connection because the topic of our illness always seems to be lingering in the air. Many do not know what to say or what to do, and the last thing a chronically sick person wants to be is a burden on those very people who had provided all that support over the years before we were the sick person. I struggled with this then, and I continue to struggle with it. My illness became more of my identity than anything else I had ever done or accomplished in my life. And that was unfair. I became the woman with a brain tumor. I was the woman who had had brain surgery. I was the friend or colleague who was going for radiation. At any social event, people would ask how I was feeling, what was the update, could they do anything for me. Some avoided me because they did not know what to say. But I wanted to just be free to be me and not be my illness nor my experience. I wanted to be appreciated for who I was as a human, a mother, a friend, and a neurologist, and for the things I *still* wanted to accomplish in life. The tumor was like a chain tied to my ankle keeping me in the same place.

I was at home alone much of this time because my husband had returned to work and our daughter was back in school. I was still unable to chew without significant pain, I was losing weight, I still had staples in my skull from ear to ear, and I felt terrified about what was to come. Every day. It was hard to articulate my feelings to my husband or my friends because I wanted so badly for things to feel normal in my home and in my life.

Adding to my feelings of isolation and disconnect was the fact that my husband was often bouncing around the house, seemingly giddy and happy and in a great mood, while I was lying there in pain. Finally I couldn't stand it anymore. "How can you be so cheerful?" I asked. It even hurt to talk. His answer seems obvious in retrospect, but at the time it walloped me. He said that for the seven and a half hours I was in surgery, he didn't know if I was going to come out. But I did, and he was happy. I felt a lot less disconnected after that. And I fell in love with him all over again.

Over time, the details of my story became less known to others, and then, over time, there was a different experience. At present, I still, on some days, struggle with fatigue, headaches, and nausea. But now, I meet many people on a regular basis who are not familiar with my medical history, and it is more of an invisible illness.

People see me as healthy, without concern, and just caring for others who are not healthy. People see me as having as much energy as the day is long and do not hesitate to ask me to do things that would easily drain my finite reserve. People would often not guess that today is a bad day for me. So, while my diagnosis is very different from those of my patients, the overall experience is somewhat similar.

Seeing and Listening

SINCE MY TUMOR WAS NOT diagnosed soon enough, it had invaded part of my brain, and the surgeon had had to scrape out some brain tissue when removing it. Later, smaller tumors would return, and I would undergo cyberknife radiation to treat them—and to this day I still have post-traumatic episodes about those treatments, during which I was bolted to the table in a mask so my head would not move—but for now I recovered. Slowly, slowly. I did a lot of juicing of vegetables and fruit to get nutrition without having to aggressively use my chewing apparatus. My jaw muscles reconnected, and I began to eat real food. The first solid meal I ate was miso mush-room tofu soup. I'll never forget the mild pain and fear that I'd re-tear the muscles but also the pure joy as the miso flavor filled my mouth and sank into my stomach. My pain decreased week by week.

Soon, my thoughts turned to my medical practice. Before the surgery, I had been planning to open my own neurology practice, and in fact I already had a space that would have to be built out, though I'd had to halt construction while going through treatment. Now it was time to get work going again and to think about my own approach to medicine. I thought about how I'd spent a year not being listened to when I expressed not only my symptoms but my anxieties over these symptoms, and I knew I was not alone in that experience. I felt a sense of urgency to help others, and I realized that with my own practice, I could do that. Like most doctors, I went into medicine because I wanted to help people, and I was a good doctor, but I wanted to do better. That was why I'd done the integrative medicine classes and fellowships—I was doing what I thought I could do. But now I would have the autonomy to give patients more time and more consideration. I would look them in the eye instead of staring at a computer screen, and I would truly listen to them. Every patient has a story, and understanding that story requires details from the patient.

Thinking about the future in this way gave me new energy and hope. And motivation. It's a funny thing about life: Realizing I had more of it behind me than I did in front of me created a deep resolve to do what I could for my fellow humans that was almost blinding—in a good way.

I did not know yet that I would come to specialize in post-exposure illnesses (PEIs) and the mysterious, chronic symptoms they create, but I was on my way. The roadway was paved and ready. Because while cancer is not as controversial a diagnosis as are post-exposure illnesses, I knew what it was like not to be taken seriously, to be dismissed, just as patients with PEIs often are. I knew what it was like to know your body is telling you something, only for others to suggest it is telling you nothing. I also know what it is like to suffer from something for which there is no consensus as to why it occurred in the first place. PEIs can seem unreal and obscure, but they are not. They're very real, and I would learn all about them soon enough, just by sitting and listening to my patients for as long as it took to find out.

As for the letter I wrote to my daughter—she never read it. But at her bat mitzvah two years after my surgery, I read it to her during the ceremony. I held the paper in my trembling hands, and I could not stop my voice from quivering. I had to stop several times to compose myself and take a breath. My husband put his arm around me to let me know he was there. I recall hearing my mother sob. I was overcome with emotion. It clearly resonated, as there was not a dry eye in the house.

I read about my love for her: "You are a bright light with a lot to offer this world, and nothing would make me prouder than for you to live as you are today: kind, generous, authentic, happy, and compassionate. Having you was by far the greatest joy of my life, and for that I am grateful."

I read to her things I had learned and wanted her to know: "Life can be hard, but we show up. If we can show up for the easy parts, we can show up for the hard parts."

And I read to her this line, which was already an important part of my life's philosophy but would, in the months and years to come, become a guiding principle of my work and my life: "Never stop being curious. Almost everything is so much more interesting when you go beneath its surface."

And my daughter hugged me tighter that day.

2

Normal, Then Sick, Then Not Normal

I OPENED MY PRACTICE ABOUT eight months after surgery, and I will never forget my first patient. Danielle was in her early thirties, a professional dancer who had been having a lot of different symptoms involving just about every organ system, including joint pain—which she attributed to dancing—food intolerances, skin issues including hives, swelling in her hands and feet, headaches, dizziness, and neck pain. She could not turn her head to the right, because she felt like she'd pass out if she did. She had problems with her gastrointestinal system and her menstrual cycle. She'd been to several specialists before me, including another neurologist. She was no closer to understanding the reason for her symptoms, and worse yet, she felt invalidated and dismissed. One of the physicians even attributed her food intolerances to an eating disorder based on nothing more than the fact that she was a dancer.

Danielle began to cry as she described all this to me. Her face contorted with pain, and in my effort to listen and make her feel seen, I refused to look away. I scribbled notes on a pad without breaking eye contact with her, which has since become my default approach. (Later, I will have to decode these often sloppy scribbles.) In medical school, we're trained to ask yes/no questions, but instead I also asked open-ended questions and gave her the time and grace to tell her story.

I could give her that time, of course, because I had lots of it—my schedule was not remotely full. My new practice was not busy yet, and though I knew it would not be that way forever, I took advantage of the opportunity to ask her lots of questions, including life story questions. What did she enjoy as a kid? Did she have limitations in terms of her activity as a kid? Had she had any surgeries, or was she ever hospitalized? Was she ever in a motor vehicle accident? Did she have allergies? Did she ever have any pain disorders such as headaches or stomachaches? Did she have any falls or concussions? How were her sleep, her appetite, and her elimination—both urination and defecation? Did she feel like she kept up with other kids physically and cognitively? Was she a happy child, and did she feel she was a healthy child? Did family members have similar symptoms to hers? When did she have her first period? Then I went on to ask about her college years. I asked what her relationships were like, whether they were traumatic, and whether she had any lingering physical or emotional feelings about them. I asked neurological questions, such as did she ever feel any numbness, tingling, or radiating pain or weakness. Did she ever experience double vision or loss of vision? Could she swallow easily and breathe easily? Did she choke a lot? Did she have chest pain? I asked about her likes and dislikes, who was in her life, who had been in her life, and who did she hope to be. Who had she hoped to be when she was twelve? Did she enjoy doing what she did?

As you can probably tell, I did not have much of a plan. I was just trying to get to know her, searching for needles in a haystack. Anything to grasp on to that might shed light on Danielle's unusual constellation of symptoms. She must have been shocked that I was spending so much time with her and asking so many questions, especially after so many doctors had seemed so rushed. And, though it took all that time, I did start to figure some things out. I learned that she'd had a lot of knee and ankle pain in her life, and she had frequently rolled her ankle playing sports when she was young. She'd gone to physical therapy several times as a teen due to pain she experienced while dancing. She had ligament laxity, which means her joints were hypermobile. She would often sublux, or dislocate, her shoulder, and have to have it popped back in, and in fact she could do this at will and did it for me in my office. I did an exam and found that she had a very, very wide range of motion—she could do back bends with virtually no effort at all. Because she was a dancer, that didn't seem *that* unusual, but it was clearly outside of the normal realm of how a person should be able to move. I sent her to a physical therapist I knew who worked with an orthopedic surgeon who had some specialty with joint flexibility, and I asked them to work on her joint range of motion. They were able to stabilize her spine, and her back pain improved.

I also noticed that she was very sensitive to things—she had a sensitive constitution and was vulnerable to different exposures, such as to food, particles in the air, creams she put on, the sun, even to certain clothes. She would get rashes easily, and she had eczema, allergies, and asthma, which is referred to as the triad. I started her on antihistamines, and that helped with those symptoms.

I conducted a bunch of diagnostic examinations, including labs, and found that she had hypothyroidism, which had not been picked up by previous labs because nobody had run a full thyroid panel, and which was likely causing her overall body weakness, problems with her menstrual cycle, hair loss, changes in her skin and nails, and bloating. I prescribed her levothyroxine for that, which helped with those symptoms. I also found that she had a vitamin B12 deficiency, which was likely responsible for symptoms of tingling as well as feelings of sadness, and I got her on B12 supplements. I ordered an MRI of her head and neck, which showed she had a straightening of her cervical spine, which at that time was thought to be solely due to muscle spasms around the spine. I put her on muscle relaxants, which helped with her back pain. Her blood pressure was low in the clinic, and because of her reported bouts of lightheadedness, dizziness, and feeling like she was about to pass out, I put her on a commonly used medication called fludrocortisone, which expands the plasma volume by retaining sodium and which helped alleviate those issues. I talked to her about integrative approaches to gut health to address what had previously been diagnosed as irritable bowel syndrome (but which I now know was mast cell activation disorder, a condition I will discuss further in the next chapter), and I got her on marshmallow tincture, glutamine supplements, and licorice tincture. I referred her to other specialists to help her with joint pain and racing heart.

My approach with Danielle was haphazard and slow—I saw her several times for hours at a time—but it eventually led to success. When she saw me a few months later for a short follow-up, she was feeling a lot better. All it took was a doctor who would listen to her. And who had lots of time, of course.

The World of Complex Illness

IN THOSE FIRST FEW MONTHS at my practice, I of course saw patients with more typical, or common, neurological issues—issues that can be scary and complicated, but that are well understood and for which we have an obvious path for treatment. But I also started to see more patients like Danielle, who over a long period of time had been experiencing a broad range of symptoms that did not coalesce into any obvious illness, injury, or condition. Word of mouth was getting out that I was giving these patients time, and I was figuring out how to help them. I was getting a good reputation, and doctors were referring their patients with complex illnesses to me.

As time went by, I honed my approach. It was still time-consuming, and it still usually took several visits, but I started to understand what I was looking for, and so I was able to sharpen my questioning and zero in on responses that I knew were meaningful. When patients first came to me, I'd start asking questions as indicated by their symptoms, and by their third or fourth visit, I would have an epiphany, which would be incredibly rewarding. Soon, I was deeply engaged in the world of complex illness. I was using everything at my disposal to treat these patients, including conventional approaches and integrative approaches. It felt good. It felt like I had found something I had long been looking for.

I started my career very much as a conventional neurologist, but along the way I started to feel a sense that what I was doing was not enough. It *was* enough in all the standard ways in which we were trained: When I saw a patient with this symptom I would do this workup, and this diagnosis would be treated with this drug or with that drug. But often, patients were not getting better, and they would return for follow-up appointments with the same symptoms, sometimes worse, often accompanied by new symptoms. I would increase the dose of the first medication I tried or switch to a different medication. But I was frustrated. Now, I was still getting frustrated, but I was channeling my frustration into better care. By the time the patient returned for the third or fourth appointment and they were not significantly better, I would go back to the beginning and ask many of the same questions but with more follow-up inquiry now that I had known them longer and understood better what their body did and did not respond to. And I would listen. Again. Harder. I found myself synthesizing other hypotheses in my head that I had not considered previously because they were not part of the "standard of care," which is what is taught and trained during medical school and residency years and then even more firmly fixed during practice and at conferences.

Initially, I did not fully trust my suspicions, because I was firmly entrenched in imposter syndrome. Who was I to see things differently when there were many minds, way smarter than mine, who had seen similar patients with similar presentations? I could not fathom how I might see things any differently than they did. But I did. I began to trust myself more and more and started to firmly connect the pieces of each patient's puzzle. Almost always, those puzzle pieces took me outside of neurology, and I found myself reading the literature of other specialties to get some understanding of the delicate and intricate interactions between the cells of different organs and between different organs and different systems.

Over the years, I have improved my diagnostic skills greatly, though I have certainly not yet perfected what I do. My education has been exponential, and even now there is not a month that goes by that I don't learn at least one new thing. In fact, I learn new things all the time. Even so, now that I have learned to recognize repeatable complex constellations of symptoms, there are times when a patient will say very little before I already know so much about what is going on with them. But I give everyone the time and respect they deserve to tell me what they want to tell me. Because there is always something interesting or intriguing to hear.

As a side note, my diagnostic workup very commonly includes a wide array of labs, which in our American healthcare system is typically considered a waste of resources. Few things irk me more than that kind of thinking. A waste of resources? The insurance-based models that most hospitals and their administrations subscribe to put up roadblocks and obstacles, but suffice it to say that ordering some extra labs and imaging is not nearly the waste of resources that occurs in just about every other facet of healthcare. The complexities of why symptoms develop and persist and why suffering exists are beyond a simple panel of tests. Frankly, advances in medicine have given us the ability and the competence to look for anatomical and physiological aberrations in patients, so why would we not take advantage of that in an effort to relieve human suffering? Because the bean counters at hospitals and insurance companies deem it a waste of resources? Doctors are intelligent humans who obviously have succeeded through many years of schooling and training, yet

healthcare bureaucrats show little respect for our analysis, our consideration, our hypotheses, and our time. We
are constantly questioned, and that's especially true for
those of us who treat complex and chronic illnesses that
are not well understood or are downright controversial. At
any rate, I see complex patients, and that requires a wide
breadth of testing. The patient deserves that.

Understanding Post-Exposure Illness

MOST PATIENTS WITH COMPLEX AND chronic illness
have at least five diagnoses, and many have more. This may
sound alarming; it was to me, initially. I used to think it
was unusual when I saw a patient with so many diagnoses. Conventionally, a person will have a single diagnosis
that may be associated with several symptoms, but those
symptoms do not change the core diagnosis. For example,
a diagnosis of Parkinson's disease includes symptoms such
as tremors, slow movements, change in gait, and change
in how the patient's face looks, but they still have the diagnosis of Parkinson's disease, and the treatment offered
is the accepted treatment for that diagnosis. And that still
holds true in a very conventional sense.

For better or worse, chronic and complex illness does
not suit the conventional definitions of diagnosis. And the
deeper I went with my patients, and the more I recognized
how the body and all its parts are truly interconnected and

how many diseases can have a multitude of downstream and upstream effects, it became clear that multiple diagnoses are not uncommon, and perhaps these diagnoses are really just subheadings under one big umbrella disease, which I have come to think of as post-exposure illness (PEI). The different diagnoses do provide somewhat of a map to decide how best to start and monitor treatment.

The multitude of symptoms is what makes PEIs so difficult to understand and what can potentially turn many doctors in the wrong direction. When complex and chronically ill patients with diagnoses that are not yet well understood and sometimes ineptly named, as in "chronic fatigue," do not respond to a few medications—or, worse, have adverse effects from them—doctors will often reflexively, and somewhat defensively, decide their symptoms are not real or at least are no longer worth trying to treat. Many doctors are uncomfortable with not knowing or with practicing in a space of uncertainty, and a defense mechanism (whether conscious or unconscious) is to assume it must be the patient's fault. In neurology, we often see patients whose symptoms don't respond to a multitude of medicines we try. We call these *refractory* disorders, as in refractory headaches or refractory epilepsy. In labeling them that way, we are implicitly acknowledging that the symptoms are real. We do not label these patients as psychosomatic or refer them to psychiatry. I have come to understand that what we see as refractory is really a symptom for which we have not found the true cause and therefore have not yet offered the appropriate treatment. And while we understand many of these refractory symptoms, by and large, we don't understand PEIs.

So what are post-exposure illnesses? How are people getting them? In a nutshell, your body is exposed to something, such as a virus, and it has a reaction to that. You get sick. Then you get better, but you don't *totally* get better. Your body has changed because of that infection, and you experience symptoms on an ongoing basis. These symptoms can be the same for a long time, and some may get better, but some may get worse. And new symptoms may appear. And what can be frustrating is you see different doctors, and they all have different ideas and different recommendations.

Besides viruses, other exposures that can trigger a PEI include bacteria, mold, environmental toxicants and contaminants, food, medications, and more. You can get a PEI after having mononucleosis or strep throat, after breathing the dust of lead paint, after taking a medication prescribed by your doctor, after eating a bad egg salad sandwich, from animal scratches, or from a tick that transferred the bacterium that causes Lyme. As most of us know now, exposure to a coronavirus such as SARS-CoV-2, the virus that causes Covid-19, can lead to a PEI we call Long Covid. It all comes down to our immune system and how it responds to exposures. Each one of us has our unique immune response, and it is shaped by our genetics and our environment—the things we have been exposed to in our lives. Because we are unique, our reaction to different exposures can be different. The new field of "omics" is teaching so much about how truly individualized our immune cells and responses are. We are on the verge of knowing so much more about why one person is vulnerable and another isn't.

The most feared exposure is to viruses. We are now learning that diseases that we have studied for decades may have their origins in viral exposures. This includes multiple sclerosis and Alzheimer's disease. Though familiar to neurologists, less well-known diseases, such as Guillain-Barré syndrome (GBS), chronic inflammatory demyelinating polyradiculoneuropathy (CIDP), febrile infection-related epilepsy syndrome (FIRES), acute demyelinating encephalomyelitis (ADEM), and transverse myelitis (TM), have long been known to follow an infectious period, which can include a very mild illness. When a patient presents with symptoms of any of these diagnoses, one of the first things we ask is if they have had a recent illness. It is scary to think that catching a cold could possibly lead to something more dire, but yes—viruses are ingenious and resilient and tough. They hijack our genome and use our own innate mechanisms for replication and protein synthesis to keep themselves alive. And when they do, they wreak havoc on our cellular functions and signaling, and they can easily alter gene expression so that any variant that may be held silent in our genome now has the potential of being expressed, which can change the course of health and of disease. Our genes hold great potential to enhance or detract from our quality of life, and each and every

Common Exposures

Post-exposure illness can result from a wide variety of different exposures. Here are the most common.

VIRUSES

Epstein-Barr Virus (EBV)

SARS-CoV-2 (the virus that causes Covid-19)

Human Herpes Virus 6, 7

Herpes Simplex Virus

Cytomegalovirus

BACTERIA

Streptococcus (can cause strep throat and other illnesses)

Borrelia Burgdorferi (can cause Lyme disease)

Pet zoonoses (diseases that can jump from nonhuman to human)

TOXICANTS

Gadolinium (heavy metal)

Arsenic (heavy metal)

Lead (heavy metal)

Pharmaceutical residues (in water and other parts of the environment)

Agent Orange

Burn pit debris

MEDICATIONS

Fluoroquinolones

Antimicrobials (antibiotics, antivirals, antifungals, antiparasitics)

Chemotherapies

Immunosuppressants

OTHER

Mold

exposure—be it intentional, through choices we make in our lifestyle options, or unintentional, due to infection, illnesses, medications prescribed by trusted doctors, herbs given by well-regarded practitioners, contaminants from industry, or more—can alter them and change how they are expressed and thus change what and how much of a particular protein or enzyme is made.

While I have worked with countless patients throughout the years who have developed chronic illness as a result of some sort of exposure, the vast majority of people are able to fight off the effects and return to their baseline for health. This raises the question: Why do some people develop chronic conditions and others do not? Through my experience of talking with patients, I have noticed some common themes in those who do develop PEIs. Many tell stories of catching mono in high school or college that put them in bed for three months. Many have a history of rashes, eczema, asthma, or allergies (and often all four). I did not quite understand it yet when I was asking Danielle, the dancer, all those questions about her younger years, but that has become standard practice for me now, because it is always illuminating. These patients often report frequently being sick as a kid, and often taking lots of antibiotics as a result. They were exposed to different organisms ("bugs"), and then they were exposed to lots of antimicrobial pharmaceuticals. Many times, I have heard patients talk about a childhood spent going to doctors as their parents tried to figure out their allergies or their sore joints or their stomach pains or their headaches, so much so that the kid would be begging to just let it go. Can we just stop going to the doctor? At some point, they did stop going to the doctor, as no one seemed to know how to help.

The Five Categories of Dysfunction

WHAT THESE PATIENTS HAVE IN common is an immune system that was on active alert for a long time. When that happens, it can make us more vulnerable to exposures in the future because, in essence, our threshold and tolerance for resiliency against these exposures is lowered. This may seem illogical, since exposure is how we increase immunity. That is why we get inoculations that contain a tiny dose of a certain disease in order to stimulate the immune system to build up a stronger defense against that disease. But for some people—again, depending on their earlier exposures and genetic makeup—certain exposures can lead to this intense, prolonged response in the body, and that can set them up for future PEIs. In other words, it may be an early exposure or a genetic variant within our genome that makes us vulnerable, and a later exposure that causes the chronic condition. We sometimes refer to this as a two-hit hypothesis, where the first hit is the initial exposure or the variant, and then the second hit is the last exposure that then leads to the disease. Incidentally, neither the initial nor the latter exposure has to be infectious, because there is much in our environment that is just as—if not more—toxic.

Our genetics should not be dismissed as easily as "no variants identified." We all hold secrets in our genome that contribute both directly and indirectly to our health. The genes are responsible for making something that has some effect on the function of our bodies. Recently, we have found genes that contribute to the risk for all sorts of diseases even if just by changing the function of an enzyme or a protein or even the internal environment by just a little bit. We also know that all kinds of exposures—especially to infectious things such as viruses—can alter the expression of genes and any variant. So while some variants may be of "uncertain significance," the level of cumulative exposures we may have had can easily change the extent to which that gene is expressed, and, in my opinion, if the symptoms match what that gene is known to participate in, it likely does hold clinical significance. Let's unlock these doors that close us into conventional thinking so we can find answers and help each other.

Most of the symptoms of PEIs are related directly or indirectly to the body's immune response, which sounds like a simple statement, but the immune system is a complex and complicated system with many pathways and many cellular components. To make it easy to understand, the symptoms experienced by those with chronic illnesses stem from at least one of the following five diagnoses, and usually more than one, each of which is triggered directly or indirectly by the immune system.

Connective Tissue Dysfunction

Connective tissue deserves a ranking as its own organ in our body and deserves more respect for its incredibly critical role in our overall health. Of all the types of tissue found in our bodies, it is the most abundant. Connective tissue is ubiquitous in our bodies. It surrounds and holds every organ, blood vessel, bone, nerve fiber, and muscle in place. It lines our mucosal membranes such as the gastrointestinal tract and the respiratory tract, it lines our hollow organs such as our bladder, and it lines the outside of our blood vessels. Our lymph and our blood are connective tissues. Connective tissue encloses and protects our brain and spinal cord, makes up our bones and tethers them to muscles, and holds our joints together, including our vertebral joints. It even holds the adipocytes (fat cells) together to form a solid layer of fat tissue.

Connective tissue does not only hold things in place, either. It is more than just a structural and mechanical organ (though that is obviously an important job). It also is very much a part of the overall body functioning. Connective tissue is a harbor for lots of activity, including a place for exchange of oxygen, nutrients, and information between our various systems. In fact, blood is a specialized type of connective tissue, whose function is to transport oxygen, nutrients, and waste by-products. Fascia, the thin casing of connective tissue that surrounds and holds every organ, blood vessel, bone, nerve fiber, and muscle in place, has nerves that make it almost as sensitive as skin. When stressed, it tightens up (which is why many patients feel some relief with fascial release work).

It helps to think of the human body as a cohesive network of tissues. I don't see patients as only their central nervous system or their peripheral nervous system or their autonomic nervous system—I see them as a holistic, cohesive network of tissues that communicate with one another and work with one another for overall support of physiology. Holding it all together is connective tissue.

Because connective tissue is everywhere in our bodies, and because it supports the overall function of all body tissues, you can see how a connective tissue disorder can wreak havoc. I often think the dislocations and the subluxations of the joints due to ligamentous laxity is like the canary in the coal mine. To begin with, the location of each individual anatomical component in your body is genetically predetermined—our parts have places where they are supposed to be. So when, due to failing or malfunctioning connective tissue, some part of the anatomy doesn't sit where it is supposed to, even if it is off by one millimeter, the cells within our bodies have trouble signaling one another. For the most part, this doesn't pose a huge problem, but over time it potentially can, as the signals consistently get lost or dropped, and therefore the organs don't communicate as well and then do not function as a whole. It is like calling for your friend who you think is on the corner, but she never comes to you because she is actually around the corner so she does not hear you calling for her.

Connective tissue is made of collagen fibers as well as

other materials, including different types of cells such as macrophages (a type of white blood cell), stem cells in different states of differentiation, cells of the immune system, and mast cells. In fact, connective tissue contains a very high concentration of mast cells, which are our first responders at the slightest hint of an attack. We will discuss them in greater detail soon, but for now know that when they are activated for prolonged periods of time, along with activated macrophages—another first responder type of cell—they can contribute to an inflammatory state in the tissue. The connective tissue becomes inflamed and can eventually begin to degrade, largely due to many of the pro-inflammatory mediators released by the mast cells, including enzymes that target the collagen layers of connective tissue for destruction. The inflammation and erosion can put patients at greater risk for all sorts of problems, including more joint subluxations; joint dislocations; spinal instability; diffuse pain of the joints, muscles, and nerves; and more.

It can also lead to distinct anatomical diagnoses such as craniocervical instability (CCI), in which the joint where the brain meets the spine has too much mobility, which can cause all sorts of symptoms such as bad headaches, chronic fatigue, low blood pressure when standing, dizziness, balance problems, vision problems, swallowing problems, neck and face pain, sleep apnea, and more; a tethered spinal cord, in which the spinal cord is pulled down and stuck on the wall of the spinal canal and can't move freely, resulting in pain, bladder dysfunction, worsening of CCI symptoms; and myriad other anatomical diagnoses. As we learn and treat an ever-increasing number of patients who have experienced infectious and other noxious exposures that created both an aberrant immune response but also other underlying diseases that further make the connective tissue "sick," we see more anatomical misalignment problems such as compressions of veins and arteries. These vessels deliver oxygenated blood to organs and take away deoxygenated blood. But if a vein is compressed, then it is like the closed exit on a highway: Everything just backs up, gets congested, and road rage happens. Anatomical diagnoses usually cause tremendous disability and commonly require surgical intervention for correction.

Like Danielle, many PEI patients are hypermobile, and some have Ehlers-Danlos syndromes (EDS), a hereditary disease that affects the connective tissue in just about every organ system in the body, particularly the joints, skin, and blood vessels. EDS can lead to problems with the collagen and can cause loose joints, joint pain, very stretchy skin, and other symptoms. People with EDS may bruise easily and not heal well from injuries. It is important to note that there are more than thirteen different subtypes of EDS, and the genetic variants for them have been identified. But the hypermobile type of EDS has been somewhat elusive, and we have not yet found the genetic variant responsible. It is possible it is caused by more than one gene. It is also possible it is nongenetic but acquired, meaning due to chronic inflammatory states from exposures. Sometimes we refer to it as hypermobility spectrum disorder.

Lax ligaments will only worsen with aging and without management, leading to poor joint stabilization that can develop into pathological anatomical conditions that increase suffering. The craniocervical joint is held together by many ligaments, because it houses critical anatomy such as the lower part of the brain stem and arteries that feed the brain its blood and veins that drain the brain, as well as compartments where cerebrospinal fluid flows. When that joint becomes unstable, it can cause compression of these contents, which can cause headaches, autonomic dysfunction, facial pain, difficulty swallowing and talking, increased intracranial pressure, abnormal visual function, pulsatile tinnitus (ringing of the ears), radiating sensory symptoms down arms and legs, and more. This is just one of several disorders that can be caused by connective tissue dysfunction in and around the brain, brain stem, and spinal cord. But it can be the most disabling because of the symptoms associated. Importantly, when blood and cerebrospinal fluid cannot flow freely, the glymphatic system of our brain— which functions to "cleanse" our brain of the debris and waste products of everyday functioning—does not work as well, as it relies on fluid flow. This waste can build up in the central nervous system, only contributing to the inflammation of the brain that patients already are experiencing.

Mast Cell Activity

Mast cells are ubiquitous cells present throughout our bodies at different concentrations in each organ system. As an integral part of our innate immune system, they are our first responders when our barriers are breached by an infectious organism, a toxic substance, a contaminant, or even a physical trauma, poised to attack at the body's slightest request. Our mast cells are situated in perfect locations throughout the body: the respiratory tract, the salivary glands, the gastrointestinal tract, the skin, and more. When our body perceives a threat, such as a virus, our mast cells activate and release hundreds of mediators—chemicals that combat the intruder, such as histamine, interleukins, prostaglandins, leukotrienes, and serotonin. Most of these mediators are already produced and stored in the mast cells and can be deployed quickly, but as the war against the virus (or whatever the exposure is) goes on, our mast cells make more of these mediators as well as other mediators to strengthen the fight. After the war is won and the exposure is eliminated, mast cells release more mediators to clean up and repair the damage from the war.

When our mast cells are activated and releasing mediators, we experience the effects of many of these mediators, as they all play a largely inflammatory role somewhere in the body. We may get headaches or stomach pains; we may feel flushed or develop rashes and itching. We may experience abdominal bloating or swelling of the hands and feet.

We may get dizzy or lightheaded, and our heart rate may go up. These are pretty much the symptoms we recognize from being sick, right? Eventually, for most of us, they go away after the mast cells and other first responder cells of our innate immune system have done their job and sense we have healed, or at least the danger is abating.

So what can go wrong? Well, this design is evolutionary from a time when our environment was cleaner, our food purer, and we did not travel as much to faraway places. We have vastly increased our exposure to things our systems may be completely naïve to. As the world has gotten dirtier, our exposures have expanded. A study done by the Environmental Working Group (EWG) in 2005 found more than 200 different contaminants in umbilical cord blood.[1] Before we're even born, we are already exposed. Industrialization and technology have pushed us to the brink, and the Environmental Protection Agency (EPA) can only do so much against the behemoth of industry lobbyists, and they are at the mercy of governmental favor, which in recent years they haven't gained. Globalization has taken us to farther places, and it has also brought faraway places closer to us.

As I mentioned, while getting my PhD in environmental toxicology, my dissertation topic was pharmaceutical residues in the waters of our country. I chose this topic

---

1 Environmental Working Group, "Body Burden: The Pollution in Newborns," July 14, 2005, https://www.ewg.org/research/body-burden -pollution-newborns.

because I always suspected our environment was making us sick, or at least putting us at greater risk of becoming sick, and because as a physician I was prescribing medications every day, and I felt I was part of the supply chain of medications journeying from the pharmacy to the environment. I found that our water does indeed contain trace amounts of just about every class of medication that exists, including antibiotics, antidepressants, antihypertensives, anxiolytics, opiates, and more. Our water technology is not yet advanced enough to filter these molecules out before they come out of our tap. I learned of the many ways in which unused pharmaceuticals find their way into the environment—usually by being flushed down toilets or poured down the sink, and sometimes through disposal in the garbage where they end up in landfills and leach into the soil. But we also urinate and defecate some of these medications and/or their metabolites as well as wash off topical medications in our showers and baths. For my research, I was working as a contractor for the U.S. EPA and had the tremendous and rewarding opportunity to work with some of the best environmental scientists in our country, who taught me that the prognosis for our environment with which humans regularly interact is dire. Even though we are talking about parts per trillion, which may not seem like a lot, remember that we are also talking about the effect of cumulative exposures over decades of life. We know from research that species that rely on water systems for life, such as fish and amphibians, suffer physiological damage from exposure to contaminants. It's logical that it would affect us, too. And sure enough, that is what research is finding. Referred to as the exposome, environmental triggers such as food additives, air pollution, and toxins from agriculture are proving to have at least some contribution to neurodegenerative disease.

The bottom line is that we are, more than ever before in our evolution, exposed and vulnerable to infections, contaminants, and toxicants. And our bodies cannot keep up.

But our immune system, starting with our mast cells, really does try. And over time, with continued exposure assault, the mast cells can get stuck and become hypervigilant, super sensitive and easily triggered, and they don't really know when to stop. They perceive danger everywhere, and they lose the ability to read the signals that tell them that there is no longer danger present, that they can calm down, and that everything is fine. With chronic activation of the mast cells, we experience chronic and systemic inflammation, which leads to a variety of possible symptoms, including pain, fatigue, swelling, itching, tingling, bloating, headaches, dizziness, elevated heart rate, and more. We are born with a built-in stopgap of any inflammatory response. But with chronic activation of immune response cells from a multitude of cumulative exposures over the years, that stopgap signal is lost in the haze.

Those with chronically overactive mast cells may be diagnosed with mast cell activation syndrome (MCAS), and they are lucky if they are, because it means the doctor who diagnosed MCAS will understand the diagnosis and know how to begin to treat its symptoms. But overactive mast cells can cause a lot more trouble for our bodies. In fact, as the primary foot soldiers in our bodies' battles against infection, imbalance, and disease—and even if just perceived—they are the linchpin that sparks and connects much of the dysregulation and ultimately the symptoms connected to PEIs, as you will see.

As I mentioned earlier, there is a high concentration of mast cells within connective tissue, and their activity within connective tissue disrupts the function of the gastrointestinal tract, leading to problems with movement of waste products, a condition known as dysmotility. Dysmotility can cause nausea, vomiting, diarrhea, bloating, constipation, and other symptoms. Dysmotility can become severe, and many will develop gastroparesis, which is significantly delayed gastric motility. Once movement of the tract slows down, waste becomes stagnant, and the microbiome becomes unhealthy and imbalanced. Compounds produced by an unhealthy microbiome can then have an unhealthy relationship with the immune system and the nervous system.

Another potential problem that can result from overactive mast cells in the GI tract—and which is related to the stagnation from slow motility—is dysbiosis, a problem with the diversity of the gut bacteria. Dysbiosis can cause abdominal pain or burning, bloating, vomiting, and more. Patients will often describe difficulty in tolerating a particular food because it causes some of these symptoms, and so they may develop a very restricted food repertoire, which can put them at risk of developing nutritional deficiencies. They are often told they are allergic to a food, but it is not actually an allergy in the true definition of the word but rather is due to the breakdown of the gastrointestinal lining and the mast cells activating within it. An angry gastrointestinal lining and the resulting problems interfere with the process of metabolizing even the healthiest of meals, which can result in feeling like you are just not able to tolerate that particular food (and which will lead many people to go to great lengths to avoid it). Many patients develop nutrient deficiencies due to an inability to tolerate a variety of foods because of a mast cell response.

Additional symptoms due to the mast cell activity include irritable bladder, gastric ulcers, vasomotor dysfunction, and cerebrospinal fluid leaks from a hole in the dural layer. Clearly, this is not an exhaustive list. If you think about all the places of the body that one can find connective tissue, you can start to imagine the resident mast cells causing a local problem and the resultant effects. The reach of abnormal mast cell activity knows no bounds.

Autoreactivity

Mast cells are part of our innate immune response, which is our first line of defense against pathogens (microorganisms, such as a virus or bacterium, that can cause disease).

The job of the innate immune response is to jump into action quickly and prevent the spread of foreign pathogens in the body. It is nondiscriminatory and nonselective and will fight every invading force. A little slower to the scene is a second immune response, our adaptive immune response. Whereas the innate immune response is nondiscriminatory, the adaptive immune response is more specific to a given pathogen. When it recognizes a pathogen, it begins creating antibodies that are designed to fight that particular pathogen. While the adaptive immune response takes a bit longer, its effect is long-lasting. Those antibodies remember the pathogen and automatically kill it any time it shows up, which is why vaccines work. You get a small dose of this year's influenza virus, and your adaptive immune system fights it off and remembers how to fight that flu bug if it shows up again.

If a person has overactive mast cells that are persistently releasing inflammatory mediators, and hence causing perpetual inflammation, there is eventually damage to the cells and breakdown of those cells. This creates cellular debris—fragments of our own cells, isolated and alone, floating freely within our bloodstream. The adaptive immune system—which is always watching and waiting—gets a whiff of this debris and perceives that something is amiss. The adaptive immune system is not sure what to make of this debris, but it prefers to keep the body safe and clean if it can, so it creates antibodies to deactivate or destroy them. The problem lies in the fact that these fragmented pieces of cells came from the cells of our own body. So when the adaptive immune system creates an army of these antibodies to seek out their target, they recognize these fragments wherever they are. They recognize the fragments that are floating alone in the bloodstream and also when they are within their larger structure of the cell, and they attach and attack in much the same fashion. The result is autoreactivity—our antibodies attacking our own cells. Autoreactivity, if chronic and persistent, can increase the risk for and potentially lead to an autoimmune disease from the stress of continual antibody production against components of your own cells.

When I see patients who report symptoms such as weakness, sudden neurological symptoms that are seizure-like, or discrete symptoms like dry eyes, dry mouth, a limb that is susceptible to fatigue, or muscle and joint pain, it is likely that autoreactivity is at fault. Some patients with autoreactivity may develop an autoimmune disease that attacks the central nervous system (the brain and the spinal cord) such as multiple sclerosis or Sjogren's syndrome; that attacks the peripheral nervous system (the nerves and muscles of our body) such as myasthenia gravis or chronic inflammatory demyelinating polyradiculoneuropathy (CIDP); or that attacks the musculoskeletal system (muscles, tendons, ligaments, and bones) such as ankylosing spondylitis or rheumatoid arthritis. It is important to note there is no evidence that definitively states that autoreactivity leads to autoimmunity—they are two distinct processes. But I think it is important to treat any chronic and overarching reactivity that is a marker of immune system dysregulation.

Small and Large Fiber Neuropathies

Mast cells are everywhere, including hanging close to our sensory nerve fiber endings. Our peripheral nervous system is made up of both large fibers and small fibers, many of which are covered with a myelin sheath that acts as an electrical insulator and helps messages travel along the nerves much faster. When we have overactive mast cells causing inflammation in the body, it can begin to wear down the myelin of our large fibers, just as it does with connective tissue. Breakdown products of the myelin protein can further trigger mast cells. When the myelin is broken down, signals that are sent along the nerves don't travel very efficiently, and after a while they don't arrive at their end point at all. This disease is known as chronic inflammatory demyelinating polyneuropathy, and it is one of the more common large fiber neuropathies seen in post-exposure patients. It causes numbness and tingling and abnormal pain sensations of the limbs, usually starting in the legs.

Even more common in post-exposure illnesses is small fiber neuropathy, which includes myelinated fibers as well as unmyelinated fibers. The small fibers are pain fibers, so a lot of the time patients will describe pain in their limbs, often electrical shock–like pain, burning, stinging, or numbness. It's often patchy, just by the nature of the distribution of the small fibers, but it too can present first in the legs. The pain can wax and wane based on many factors that change the inflammatory response, such as energy state, sleep, nutritional status, stress levels, and overall health.

Small fibers also play a role in our autonomic system, so small fiber neuropathy can cause a lot of swelling and redness in the hands and feet because small fibers control how our blood vessels dilate or restrict. If they're not working very well, then you experience vasomotor dysregulation—you have dilated vessels and lots of fluid buildup. It's usually seen in the hands and feet because they are the farthest point from the trunk of our body. The small fibers also play a role in the movement of the gastrointestinal tract to move foodstuffs and digestive products through the tract. Small fiber neuropathy can contribute to dysmotility, which causes further GI symptoms as described previously.

Small fiber neuropathy is diagnosed with a skin biopsy because small fibers are close to the very edges of our skin. On the biopsy, the pathologist identifies what is called low intraepidermal nerve density, which just means you do not have enough small fibers because they have presumably degenerated due to the inflammation in your body. That can be due to autoreactivity, mast cell activity, direct invasion of pathogens, and altered glucose metabolism such as in diabetes and other metabolic and endocrine disorders. When small fiber neuropathy is diagnosed, a full workup for causes should be done, as there may be a treatable cause.

Autonomic Dysfunction

The small fibers play a role in controlling our autonomic functions, not only of the gastrointestinal tract but also our sweat glands and how we sweat, how our heart beats, and how our lungs breathe. These are the things our bodies just do—we don't have to think about them. But PEI patients often report symptoms related to dysfunction of the autonomic nervous system, such as chronic constipation or gastroparesis, which means everything is just stuck—waste is not being removed, and that can lead to an overgrowth of disease-causing microorganisms in the digestive tract. Or they may experience elevated heart rate or temperature dysregulation, the latter of which can spike other symptoms. Something as simple as a hot shower, which we may normally take great comfort from, can cause discomfort and symptoms that can take hours if not days to resolve. Or any minimal exercise or physical activity can cause intense fatigue and a prolonged period of recovery.

The most common autonomic disorder diagnosis seen in PEI patients is postural orthostatic tachycardia syndrome (POTS), which can be very disabling for patients, who experience an elevated heart rate without exertion or with a simple change in position. If you stand up, you feel lightheaded, your heart rate spikes, and you have to sit down. POTS patients can't walk for long distances, can't stand for long periods of time, may feel lightheaded or like they will pass out, and some do pass out. There is often

further suffering in the form of headaches, vision problems, and "coat hanger pain"—pain along the upper back
and shoulders, which is thought to be due to abnormal
blood flow distribution.

Usually, the patient's blood pressure remains stable, but
if it does not, it is referred to as orthostatic hypotension.
Regardless, in POTS there is an overall orthostatic intol-
erance, which means there is an inability of the vessels to
dilate and constrict appropriately to accommodate changes
in pressure and volume of blood depending on the different positions the person transitions to. For example, when
we stand, gravity tries to take over by pulling our blood
downward to our feet. In a healthy person, the vessels will
constrict in order to keep some of that blood in the brain,
whereas the vessels in a patient with POTS or autonomic
dysregulation of any type don't constrict properly. When
these patients stand, all their blood leaves their head and
upper body and goes down to their feet. And they experience those symptoms—the dizziness, the feeling like
they're going to pass out, the lightheadedness—mainly
because there is not enough blood in the brain. The blood
pools in our lower bodies and does not return to the heart.
The heart rate will rise to compensate to try to push out
more blood. But that process does not work as it should,
because when the heart is beating too fast, it does not have
enough time to fill with enough blood, so it is basically
pumping fast for nothing. It's an uncomfortable feeling to
have your heart beating at a fast rate; it can feel like you're

having a heart attack and can cause shortness of breath and fatigue, as well as lightheadedness.

With progression of a chronic illness, this autonomic dysfunction can persist at some level for most of the patient's day, contributing to the chronic fatigue and other symptoms they feel, such as brain fog, generalized weakness, headaches, difficulty breathing, and disproportionate sweating. And it can be bad. Some patients cannot get out of bed, or even be upright at all, day after day. A few develop autonomic seizures and are invariably told they have pseudoseizures, or functional seizures, which means the seizure events are not real in a conventional sense as seizures are thought to be an electrical aberration of the neurons of the brain. An electroencephalogram (EEG) may be negative, but there are limitations to that testing. But when I think of the systemic dysfunction by the chronic immune provocation, I can think of—and often find—reasons for neurons and glial cells to be unhappy and react in kind with what is absolutely a paroxysmal, discrete, acute-onset, and self-resolving neurological event—a definition of a seizure.

Perpetual inflammatory signals can break down the protection of our central nervous system by causing a breakdown of the blood–brain barrier. This allows for more inflammatory mediators to breach that barrier and enter our nervous system, negatively affecting our neural pathways and resulting in reduced energy and activity, reduced appetite, reduced interest in engagement either socially or occupationally, and sleep fragmentation. These kinds of symptoms are hallmarks of chronic illness and of sickness in general, yet they stem from responses that we have developed to help *fight* illness, including bacterial and viral infections. It is interesting that responses that have an evolutionary basis to help us recover from infectious illness have now evolved to responses that change the course of our lives and keep us sicker. That is a testament to the overwhelmed nature of our immune systems.

Solving Puzzles

THERE ARE CLEAR CONNECTIONS AND overlap among mast cell activity, autoreactivity, connective tissue disorder and the resultant anatomical malalignment diagnoses, small and large fiber neuropathies, and autonomic dysfunction. They do not exist in isolation, and patients with post-exposure illness will have some aspect of most of these diagnoses over time. For example, the extent to which there is CCI or tethered cord or internal jugular vein compression will greatly affect how the patient feels, presents, and suffers. The severity and the response to treatment may differ from patient to patient, but regardless, some combination of these diagnoses will be present in the patient and create vulnerability in their health. Importantly, these different pieces of the puzzle give the patient and their doctor a place to start to figure out what to do first and where to go from there, like a road map.

I have described my process of working with such patients. It's painstaking and can take a good amount of time. That's because there are a lot of different things going on, and each piece of the patient's puzzle has to be identified and dealt with. When I start to match up the pieces of a patient's suffering and connect their dots, I start to see the horizon for them. Often, I will be writing the chart notes for a patient after an appointment, and I will have an idea or an epiphany about a potential root cause. The process of matching up those puzzle pieces is different for each patient, but then again, I learn from each patient, too, and each one makes me that much more knowledgeable for the next patient. It is why I love what I do and greatly look forward to each patient appointment.

Everyone deserves a physician who will listen to them and be curious and work to solve the puzzle of their unique conditions. Until that time, there is a lot you as a patient can learn and do to help yourself. That's what Part II of this book provides.

3

The Past, Present, and Possible Long Future of Long Covid

AT SOME POINT IN THE fall of 2020, I started seeing patients with chronic illness who, as part of their histories I was gathering, would tell me they had had Covid that past spring. Invariably, they said the illness was not all that bad—they were not hospitalized, certainly. And they had recovered, or at least they'd mostly recovered. They no longer had the cough or other acute symptoms, but they did not return to their normal baseline, either. By the time I was seeing them, it had been many months since they'd had Covid, and they still did not feel normal. Many had developed food intolerances, or they felt dizzy or had headaches they could not get rid of. Most of them had fatigue, and for some the fatigue was unbearable. They could not sleep at night, they could not go back to work, they could not engage with their kids or partners. They would report going to bed at five P.M. and still not waking up refreshed. They found it hard to make decisions, hard to follow conversations, and hard to remember conversations they'd had the day before. Most commonly, patients told me that it felt like they were thinking through a fog. These people were really scared they were not going to get their life back.

By that time in my career, I had seen a lot of patients with chronic illnesses, including myalgic encephalomyelitis/chronic fatigue syndrome (ME/CFS); there clearly was some overlap in symptoms with what these patients were describing, though, interestingly, also some curious distinctions. One of the first thoughts I had was that maybe these were ME/CFS patients who were in early stages with that condition. All of the chronic fatigue patients whom I'd seen by then had had that condition for twenty years before I saw them, because neurologists and other doctors had not been able to help them or had not taken them seriously. I'd never seen anyone in the early days of chronic fatigue syndrome. Maybe this was what that looked like. (What I know now is that, while this was Long Covid and not ME/CFS, Long Covid patients are at risk for developing ME/CFS and many do progress to meet the criteria of ME/CFS.[1]) And, importantly, I now

---

1 Osman Moneer, "Long Covid, ME/CFS and the Importance of Studying Infection-Associated Illnesses," Yale Medicine Long Covid Blog, May 13, 2024, https://www.yalemedicine.org/news/long-covid-mecfs-and-the-importance-of-studying-infection-associated-illnesses.

take a much more active and intensive approach for my patients when they have an infection or learn they were exposed to something, in the hope of preventing lingering, diffuse disease and symptoms.

In any case, because of the work I'd been doing with PEIs, I was very keen on the idea that you could get an infection and not get better. In particular, I was thinking about viruses. My husband had had H1N1, or swine flu, back in 2009–2010, and he had not been able to get back to baseline, either. He could not get out of bed for almost four months. After a month he would try to sit at the dinner table with us, and within fifteen minutes he would go back to bed. He had always been very fit—he went to the gym all the time, and he was a workaholic—so it was alarming to see him inactive for so long. I was really worried about him. He lost thirty-five pounds during that time, but eventually he improved and was able to resume life at his own pace. It is weird to look at pictures of him during that year of his life. His skin looked sallow, his eyes had no life, and it is hard to recognize the person I married. He recovered. But many do not, and there has to be a reason why.

I was not diagnosing Long Covid at first. Nobody was. But then there were reports on patients who had had Covid and were now found to have small fiber neuropathy and autonomic dysfunction—usually POTS. There were several studies being done and papers being published. Within the patient histories described, these patients would also report they were now always fatigued, could not complete tasks that required even minimal exertion, felt lightheaded not only when standing but even with change of position or by standing too long or walking too long, and most began to describe "brain fog." I began to see the writing on the wall and to have an idea where this would be going. These patients had had an infection—Covid-19—and then they had developed a post-infection or para-infection or infection-associated illness. Either way, it was following their acute infection. They had the symptoms and indications of all the five categories of chronic illness described in the previous chapter: connective tissue dysfunction, mast cell activation, autoreactivity, small and large fiber neuropathies, and autonomic dysfunction.

As I stated, there are PEIs that show up directly after the acute exposure and there are many that are delayed. Long Covid seems to be a mixture. Some people do not return to a baseline after their acute infection, some do seem to recover but only to have a recurrence or a relapse after a few weeks or a few months, and some patients will develop Long Covid after the second or the third Covid-19 infection and not the first. It can be a mixed bag; it would be important to understand who is at risk of developing Long Covid, and not only who but why and when. Basically, we need to understand how much an individual's immune system can take before it just decides it cannot do it anymore and revolts or hides or turns against the body that it is supposed to protect.

Brain fog, in my opinion, is a patient experience, but it does not have a specific medical meaning in terms of a true diagnosis (that is, there is no official diagnosis code for brain fog). This often causes some consternation among clinicians, especially neurologists. It can be a struggle to grasp what the patient means when they say they have brain fog, but that can be remedied by asking the right questions. Patients will typically score well on cognitive tests but nonetheless struggle with memory, word recall, the speed and ease with which they process new information, and experience an inability to stay on task. They will say it is as if they are thinking through a fog. There are many ideas and theories about what potentially underlies the brain fog experience, and it is thought to be due to an overall lack of blood flow through the vessels of the brain. Part of this is vasomotor dysregulation, which is a hallmark of autonomic dysfunction, and means the vessels themselves do not respond to changes of volume and pressure of the fluid contained within them (that is, blood). In fact, some physicians will diagnose an immune-mediated process or an autoimmune encephalopathy, which means the immune system is causing inflammation in the brain, and therefore the brain—from the patient's perspective—is not working as it once did. But classically defined autoimmune encephalopathy is usually fraught with seizures and other symptoms that are not always associated with brain fog, because these other symptoms interfere with cognition, which can be seen on cognitive studies. Patients with post-exposure brain fog usually do not have seizures (at least not the usual kind with a focus seen in electroencephalograms [EEGs]), usually perform okay on cognitive testing, and have normal neurological exams.

There are other reasons that contribute to the brain fog experience that have a lot to do with inflammation of the vessels of the brain and inflammation of the brain overall due to infiltration of immune cells and the release of inflammatory mediators, which can result in reactivation of viruses and deposition of toxic substances. Early on, the brain fog does not cause cognitive impairment, at least not in the way we have come to think of cognitive impairment, or at least not yet. But the concern and the potential for further decline of cognitive abilities cannot be ignored, and indeed I often do a "cognitive impairment workup." There are certain lab tests that can be done. Based on clinical concerns I may also order some imaging as well as genetic tests, as there is recent evidence of certain genes holding risk for cognitive decline, but also certain genes can be protective. With the patient's agreement, I go down these routes.

But bottom line: Even though brain fog does not have a specific medical meaning or diagnosis, *that does not mean that what you are experiencing is not actually happening.* We may just need a new name, better understanding, or improved evaluation of patients with this experience as part of their chronic illness. As we learn more, and as more clinicians become curious and concerned, there will be better preventative and therapeutic care for all patients.

Problems in the Blood

YOU MAY RECALL THAT EARLY on in the Covid-19 pandemic, most health officials thought it was a respiratory disease. But eventually, research showed something else. The platelet activation that came with acute Covid led to vascular damage and, in some patients, insoluble small clots in their blood vessels. Referred to as "microclots," they seemed to be at least part of the reason for many of the symptoms. In most patients, as they recovered from the infection, their body was able to break down these small clots and return to normal. But for some patients, the small clots remained, clogging up the smaller vessels such as the arterioles and capillaries that feed the crevices of all organs, and thus began to cause damage to blood vessels and block blood flow to the organs they supplied. In some, even when there was appropriate breakdown of these small clots, the products of the breakdown—referred to as fibrin degradation products—triggered a large release of histamine from the mast cells. This led to widespread histamine-related symptoms (rash, hives, swelling, itching, fatigue, headache, dizziness, or nausea) as well as organ dysfunction, and thus a wide range of symptoms. Initially, the level of dysfunction was seemingly apparent only to the patient and not to the doctors they were seeing because the loss of organ function did not yet meet the level where testing showed anything wrong. That left the patient in a precarious position of either shrugging their shoulders and going home and dealing with their symptoms or trying to convince their doctor that something was indeed not right. I have been through the latter and, even for me, that was not easy. Being met with disbelief can be an uncomfortable place to be and, frankly, hard to get over.

Patients experiencing Long Covid symptoms would visit designated Long Covid clinics, or even just doctors who reported an understanding of the Long Covid syndrome phenomenon, with hope and expectation. These patients were being told that there was nothing wrong and that they needed some more rest, and they were often offered medication for anxiety and sleep. They were guided to return to normal life as well as to exercise. Some were referred to rehab programs or cognitive behavioral training, known as CBT, a common recommendation for disorders thought to be functional or related to stress and anxiety. The research was new and had not permeated the Long Covid syndrome medical world just yet to accommodate all the thousands of patients that were suffering. In retrospect, this is a failure, because the earlier something is identified, the better the chance of a patient to respond to interventions. Indeed, much current medical research and dialogue often focuses on early symptoms and biomarkers of many of the more commonly known neurodegenerative diseases such as Parkinson's disease, Alzheimer's, and amyotrophic lateral sclerosis (ALS), and even recently there have been reports of possible early biomarkers of multiple sclerosis: all in hope of diagnosing these dreaded disorders earlier so that patients can be treated earlier with the goal that, at the very least, progression is slowed, if not halted.[2]

After a couple months of seeing many patients with persistent symptoms following a Covid infection, I began to realize that it was not just small clots but larger ones as well. I noted an increase in stroke and heart attacks in patients who had a recent history of a Covid-19 infection—and these were young people, who are not typically vulnerable to strokes. They did not have other classic risk factors for stroke. Small clots theoretically don't cause strokes—it takes a larger clot. Small clots can coalesce and become a larger one, of course. Regardless, the contribution of the microclots to the increase in patients with stroke was not considered. The microclots may have contributed not only to risk of stroke and heart attack but also to the overall morbidity of the patient, which refers to the extent the disease state contributes to the decreased quality and functionality of life of the patient and is sometimes referred to as the burden of the disease. In neurology, when a patient has a stroke, we do a stroke workup to find out why they had it so we can try to prevent the next one. We check for diabetes and hypertension, we look to see if there is a hole in the heart where a clot can get through to the brain, we check the carotid arteries, and so on. It is a standard stroke workup we do as neurologists, regard-

---

2 Jens Kuhle and Pascal Sati, "The Role of Biomarkers in Multiple Sclerosis," Neurology Live, March 4, 2024, https://www.neurologylive.com /view/the-role-of-biomarkers-in-multiple-sclerosis.

less of age because these are treatable disorders and therefore something we do not want to miss. But the standard stroke workup on these Long Covid patients was almost always negative. Patients did not have any of these potentially treatable conditions. Other than their Long Covid symptoms, most of them were young and healthy—or at least previously healthy.

My first approach after reading the research was to try to thin out the blood in these patients, so I prescribed blood thinners and anticoagulants. They have small clots, so let's try to prevent more from forming. But the real question had always been why. Why were they developing clots? And that's what led me to start thinking about the mast cells. Mast cells do release mediators that create a milieu of inflammation, and there's nothing like massive inflammation to lead the body to form clots. Inflammation contributes to blood stagnation, where the blood is now very viscous and dense and does not flow as well, and it creates what is referred to as a hypercoagulable state. One way to say it is, the blood is just sort of hanging around with other blood, so it coagulates. It forms a clot. So, if you have overactive mast cells, as people do who are suffering from different forms of post-exposure illness, then your body is prone to making clots. In addition, as I stated, the products that come from the eventual degradation of these small clots—though the vessels are already damaged—trigger a histamine release from the mast cells, and that histamine creates a variety of systemic symptoms, many of which are reported in most post-exposure illnesses including Long Covid and ME/

CFS. Symptoms can be flushing, rash, fatigue, headaches, elevated heart rate, altered gut motility, pain, dizziness, visual disturbances, pelvic and abdominal discomfort, and neuropathy. At that point it was logical to connect these post-Covid symptoms to other post-exposure illnesses I had been seeing throughout my practice, such as ME/CFS and Gulf War illness, as well as other neurodegenerative disorders.

I started by becoming more insistent on stabilizing the mast cell activity, because the inflammation the mast cells caused was aggressive and was damaging the tissues of my patients—many of whom already had hypermobility, but some of whom developed hypermobility from the systemic inflammatory response. Inflammation changes the internal environment of the body and allows for breakdown of tissues, formation of clots, and damage to blood vessels, which further causes clots but also slowing of blood flow and weakening of the vessel walls. I worked hard to combat and reduce the inflammation and thin the blood to improve blood flow and to allow the blood to deliver crucial oxygen and nutrients to the tissues, and hopefully lessen the formation of clots. How I did this with each patient depended on the patient and their most prominent symptoms but also on what I may have seen on their lab workup, their imaging, or their physical exam. It may have included anti-inflammatory medications or medications that would suppress or modulate the immune system. It may have included medications that alter blood flow dynamics, medications that reduce the formation of clots, or medications to change the level or function of a neurotransmitter such as serotonin, dopamine, or even histamine. I would often recommend complementary treatment options to the pharmacological ones. Sometimes I was more aggressive and used a treatment called plasmapheresis, which has long been used for autoimmune neurological disorders, because my patients had evidence of symptoms that were due to the adaptive immune system being on high alert and in high drive and forming autoantibodies—which are antibodies that attack a piece of ourselves. I may have added some targeted supplements that supported what I was trying to treat, and I counseled on proper nutrition and how food can be used as medicine. I discussed sleep and sleep hygiene practices. I helped manage stress responses by teaching guided meditation and the use of adaptogenic herbs and other plant tinctures. Patients would start to improve, incrementally, day by day. But it wasn't linear. It was often like two steps forward, one step back. But most importantly, I was there for them and would tweak their plan based on their response.

The eventual plateau and the halting of progress was very upsetting to see, both for the patient and for me. It felt like I was standing at the edge of something, on a precipice, perhaps a solution was coming, but I could not yet visualize where we were going. The research seemed to always circle around conclusions or definitive ideas of how to treat. But meanwhile, patients kept on coming, because they were continuing to suffer. There were symptoms common to all, but each individual patient seemed to have a unique symptom or a unique piece of their medical history, and that was what made them stand out in my mind. I often wondered if that was a clue to the larger puzzle of Long Covid and then perhaps to all post-infectious diseases. I made sure I stayed on top of the research that was coming out about Covid so as not to miss a finding, an insight, or, even better, a eureka moment. I wanted to know as much as I could. I was willing to empirically try treatments based on a combination of research findings; other diseases I have treated; my training in neurology, mitochondrial medicine, and environmental toxicology; and the patients themselves.

In April of 2021 I went to the annual conference of the American Academy of Neurology, where I had the opportunity to learn a great deal about research that had been done by neurologists about Covid and its effects on the brain and the spinal cord. Many studies had been done in various hospitals, and these studies gave me ideas on what to test for, how to approach, and what I needed to do to help my patients. There is research to suggest a variety of mechanisms that underlie persistent disease from infection, and that includes a role of the virus and/or its parts sitting around in the tissues of the body for long periods of time—even well after we think the acute infection is over—but also a wayward immune system that has become hyperactive and disorganized as a response to the pieces of the viruses not wanting to leave and basically becoming a house guest that has long overstayed its welcome.

As a neurologist, I found this neurology and immunology research and its findings to be very much in sync with what I had known, seen, done, and learned of other post-exposure illnesses. I was able to draw upon the deep repertoire of modalities I had developed for treating them over the years. I think my experience and knowledge in environmental exposures and the effects on human health have provided me a unique understanding of how to approach and ultimately treat these patients. Addressing the clotting risk helps, as does trying to rein in the immune response, and, depending on a particular patient's symptoms, I will try other treatment options that I have used for other PEIs, which you will read about in Part II. Importantly, I just keep trying. Sometimes these things will have a benefit, and sometimes I must try something else. Communication with my patient and with other doctors working with the same patient population is key to knowing what a patient may need.

Each patient is unique, and each patient gets their own plan, and as is the case with my other PEI patients, it can take a long time to get to know them and to figure out, based on the evidence, what plan will work for them. But for all patients, the plan usually combines very conventional treatment options in terms of medications and other pharmacologic classes with some integrative approaches, such as certain supplements, hydration, exercises, meditation, oxygen therapies, food as medicine, and more. I make the plan with the patient as an active participant, and we change as we need to. Part of my workup includes a genetic evaluation because it may be one answer to the question as to why one person is so vulnerable, and another one is not so vulnerable. I often find variants that help explain at least part of what may be going on with an individual patient.

I have not found a "cure." Obviously, Long Covid still exists. But on the other hand, to say there's no cure is not totally accurate, because we treat the symptoms, and some patients start to feel better, and their symptoms can resolve. They can return to their baseline. And at that point, we can wean them off some of the medications, and assuming that they can stay at baseline, that's a pretty great outcome. I would say that we cured it for that person. Yet not everyone responds, and there is not yet a panacea or a blueprint despite how hard we try. But that ails most of medicine. There are very few treatments that work for 100 percent of patients with a disease. Migraine disease is a perfect example. There are myriad drugs that have been developed to treat migraines each year, and yet people still suffer, though many find their migraines to be much more manageable with the use of some of the medications and other management options. But not all have found relief.

Looking Ahead at the Long Covid of the Future

IN THE UNITED STATES, THE federal Covid-19 public health emergency was ended in May of 2023, but we continue to see new waves of infections in this country and worldwide. And we continue to see people developing Long Covid. Recent estimates indicate that more than 65 million people worldwide have Long Covid.[3] Because the symptoms can vary so widely from patient to patient, and because there is no biomarker—no test or swab or biologically derived indicator—that can diagnose somebody with Long Covid, it often gets missed, or dismissed, by doctors. And it often goes untreated. Worse yet, without a way to consistently diagnose the condition, it's very hard for researchers to study it and for patients to get appropriate care.

Less hopeful is a fear that has been creeping up on me these past couple years. At this point, I have seen hundreds of Long Covid patients, and my worry, based on what I have personally seen and what I have read in the research, is that at some point down the road—maybe in a couple decades and perhaps sooner—we're going to have an epidemic of neurodegenerative disorders.[4] We now know that there is an association between viruses and the development of neurodegenerative disorders such as Parkinson's disease, Alzheimer's disease, MS, and ALS, as

3 Anil Oza et al., "Long COVID Scientists Try to Unravel Blood Clot Mystery," *Short Wave*, NPR.com, May 15, 2023, https://www.npr.org/2023/05/10/1175217130/long-covid-scientists-try-to-unravel-blood-clot-mystery.

4 Jinyang Zhao, Fan Xia, Xue Jiao, and Xiaohong Lyu, "Long Covid and Its Association with Neurodegenerative Diseases: Pathogenesis, Neuroimaging, and Treatment," *Frontiers in Neurology* 15 (April 2024), https://doi.org/10.3389/fneur.2024.1367974.

well as prion diseases such as Creutzfeldt–Jakob disease (CJD) or fatal familial insomnia (FFI). In other words, these are post-exposure illnesses.

Recently I heard a lecture at a neurology symposium in which the speaker, a neurologist, described studies where researchers looked for certain biomarkers of dementia syndrome in Long Covid patients.[5] What they found was that the patients, who were young, have higher levels of biomarkers associated with dementia than patients who have a dementia syndrome diagnosis. And I have seen this in my Long Covid patients as well—at least the beginnings of cognitive compromise or during what they are describing as brain fog. This raises the grim possibility that Long Covid patients are at markedly higher risk for developing dementia, such as Alzheimer's disease. Given the number of people who have had Long Covid already, it's a terrible thought. In addition, I and the other physicians that see Long Covid patients each day can't help but remark on the increasing incidence of cancers in young people.

So, while I know we have helped a lot of Long Covid patients feel better, reduce their symptoms, and be more functional, I worry about what's churning inside their

---

5 Lecture by NYU Langone Health, "Blood Markers of Brain Damage Are Higher Over Short Term in Patients Who Have Covid-19 Than in People Who Have Alzheimer's Disease," https://nyulangone.org/news /blood-markers-brain-damage-are-higher-over-short-term-patients-who -have-covid-19-people-who-have-alzheimers-disease.

bodies. Or really, the body of anyone who has been exposed to the virus, whether they have developed Long Covid or not. Or any virus. Our knowledge of immune responses has grown exponentially; we know that there are individual immune responses, and some people enter a stage of immune dysregulation where their immune system does not know how to rein itself in. So, all exposures are suspect for initiating further chronic effects. Neurodegenerative disorders are delayed onset, but signs and even symptoms may be seen in retrospect, which is why eighteen-year-olds are not the classic demographic, so we won't know for some time if indeed SARS-CoV-2 has initiated a neurodegenerative process.

For that reason, I sometimes look for dementia biomarkers in my patients I'm particularly worried about, especially if, for example, they perform not as expected on cognitive testing or their partner expresses concern about a noted change in not only the patient's cognitive function but also their personality. Some of the markers in the research were found in cerebral spinal fluid, so I do lumbar punctures to try to identify them in my patients. Some of the markers are found in blood, so I screen for them in blood workups, and some are found in the same skin biopsies we do to check for small fiber neuropathy, so I check those. I also order PET scans, if I can get the insurance company to approve them, to assess metabolic activity. Depending on what I find, it can affect how aggressive I will be with a patient's treatment plan. I don't necessarily share my specific concerns about dementia with the patient, because to this point all I have is my own observations and conjecture about what might be coming. While I have a great deal of experience and knowledge, I do not have any real weight of evidence to support this fear, and I don't want to terrify my patients. My goal is to give them hope. But at the same time, we know that the earlier we identify a process or a disease state, the earlier we can get intervention started, and the greater the chance of a response and improvement—and, hopefully, lessening the tide of disease. I would like to think there is no rush—as you do want to avoid hasty decisions when working in a space with lots of uncertainty and unproven theories. It can be a fine and tricky balance, and one that I think I have learned to master and navigate with respect and kindness. When you see hundreds of patients with similar histories and symptoms and even similar triggers of flares and responses to interventions, you can pick up on a pattern that may be anecdotal or empirical. But see it enough, and it starts to hold great significance if it could mean the difference in a patient's quality and ultimate enjoyment of the one life we are all given.

So I *can* give them hope because I have hope. I believe that if indicated by their diagnostic workup, and then if I treat them aggressively enough, I can help improve their symptoms and work to maintain whatever benefit they had gotten from the treatment; and if I help them pursue a healthy preventative life, I can lower their risk of developing anything further. With Alzheimer's and other neurodegenerative disorders, there are things you can do to lower your risk—it comes down to sleep, nutrition, and exercise. Studies show the better you sleep, the better your diet, the more you exercise, the lower your chance of getting Alzheimer's disease and other diseases that can afflict us later in life—though so many Long Covid patients are so young that the risk is now a lot sooner than the typical sixth or seventh decade of life. I want my patients to live a life free of disease and symptoms. They have too much to do and too much to offer the world. I used to think I want to save the world, but I now know my role is to save the people who will save the world.

4

It's *Your* Health

I OFTEN THINK BACK TO the time soon after my surgery, starting my recovery, when I was finally alone with my thoughts. I had just been discharged from the hospital and, with my husband at work and my daughter at school, I had a lot of time to think. At first, I was in denial about the state I was in. I just wanted things to be normal. Denial and suppression were a big deal in my family during my childhood, and that is what I was used to, and I guess that is where I was comfortable. Deny it and it does not exist. Oh, but it does. Suppress it and it goes away. But it doesn't. You just don't have to face it until it grows into a big, angry monster that is now a way more formidable foe.

I turned to the part of me I was comfortable with—the doctor part. If I could not face my own future and my own health as a patient, as a human being, at least I could begin to face it as a professional. Treatment for the time being was done. The tumor was removed to the best of my surgeon's ability. I was on the appropriate medications, including anti-seizure drugs. The rest, I figured, was up to me.

Now I realize I am a doctor. I am a neurologist. And I have had schooling that most have not. I recognize the advantage I may have had with regard to how I interpreted and analyzed and chose from the various options for hastening and optimizing my recovery and my healing. But I firmly believe without a lingering doubt that most of us arrive at moments in our lives when we have no choice but to take control of our health, and in some cases, take *back* control. We not only have to learn how to advocate for ourselves, but we should spend time sitting with what we are feeling—physically, emotionally, mentally, even spiritually. When we take the time to be introspective, and we connect with how our physical bodies are communicating, and assess what our reactions to those symptoms are and how they affect us on different levels—when we are alone, when we are at work, when we are at play, when we are interacting with family, friends, and so on—we develop a deeper understanding of what is amiss. Not necessarily a true diagnosis, but you can get a sense of where something is wrong, especially when you analyze what makes a particular symptom better and what makes it worse. And then—and only then—you can make better decisions on how best to manage your well-being while you wait to see your doctor. And when you see your doctor, you will be armed with valuable and important information for that appointment. The exercise to analyze a particular symptom can be empowering. It may also lead to lots of Google searching and potentially spending time going down wrong paths and rabbit holes, so it's imperative to exercise caution. Know there are no true "biohacks." There are no easy answers, and there is no magic cure for complex and chronic illness, so be wary of the promises that seem to permeate internet searches.

The information highways can be fraught with misinformation, misinterpretation, and misunderstandings. Every doctor has their own experience with patients and tends to stick with what has been shown to be helpful to their previous patients. It is not an unreasonable way to practice. But we need more dialogue among doctors who are curious and able to take on the more complex cases and share what we know, what we see, what we do, and even take risks to share some theory we devised or suspect, without fear. Some of the best ideas come outside of evidenced-based medicine. Fortunately, there are email groups of different doctors who are interested in a specific topic. My favorite is a listserv with more than four hundred doctors at the time of this writing. What is fascinating to me about being part of this group is that initially I thought it would be only about mast cells—and to be sure it mainly is—but the interests and topics of this group go way beyond that, because we all see complex patients and are trying to put pieces of a puzzle together and share what we are learning along the way. These groups are sorely needed. Healthy and respectful conversations and sharing of resources and presentation of cases should be an ongoing activity of all physicians, especially those in the chronic illness world. I also, along with my partner, David Kaufman, MD, started a podcast called *Unraveled: Understanding Complex Illness* in an effort to further educate and disseminate information. I should add that patients themselves are often a source of education, and having them be part of the dialogue would be of tremendous benefit.

What we have discussed thus far in this book can feel overwhelming and exhausting, but despite all that may be happening with us internally, there are ways we can empower ourselves to take hold of our trajectory without the reliance on our cumbersome, clunky healthcare system. What I provide in Part II of this book is sound advice from someone who is proudly an educated integrative neurologist, who is actively treating patients with complex and prolonged illness, and who is suffering from a chronic disease herself, because I too will likely never be cured.

Each one of us is an individual, and the person you are— your genetics, your family life, your stress levels, the pathogens and other things you have been exposed to in this world, the way you live your life with regard to sleep, exercise, and nutrition—can mean that some treatments work better than others, while some don't work at all. And the best person to figure out what works is you. Communication with your doctors is paramount for your continued recovery. And it should be done without fear they will drop you or, worse, not believe you.

Doing the Little Things

THE CONVENTIONAL VIEW OF MEDICINE sometimes can make it seem that healing can occur only with a pill, but the truth is we all hold some natural healing capabilities within. We maintain neuroplasticity (the ability to create or re-create our neural connections) and mechanisms for adjusting imbalances and promoting homeostasis (an equilibrium state of our body) for most of our lives. Yet to harness those processes can take time, motivation, and dedication. Doctors can place a label, or a diagnosis, on whatever our condition is, and they can even prescribe a medication, but at each person's core is an intuition of what feels off within their body—and maybe even a sense of what helps. Sometimes it takes trial and error, but when I ask a patient, "What makes that symptom better?" or "What makes that symptom worse?" they will almost always have an answer. Your intuition about your own body and what it needs is likely better than what any doctor can tell you. You don't need a medical education, because this is not about a diagnosis label or even the mechanisms and the reasons behind the symptoms. This is about knowing what your body is experiencing on a daily basis and learning about ways you can make it either more tolerable or less tolerable. Our introspection can help guide us to find a way to improve how we feel, even if only a little, and even if only for a brief time. And in fact, many of us would take even a little relief for a brief time. To be clear, I am referring to chronic and complex illnesses such as ME/CFS or Long Covid and other fatiguing illnesses. New symptoms when one was otherwise healthy should be shared with a physician so as not to delay a diagnosis that requires treatment.

I used to regularly tell my mother, who was a long-term smoker and not so silently suffered with progressive fibromyalgia, that if she stopped smoking, she would most certainly feel better. I never suggested it would cure her fibromyalgia or offer complete resolution of her symptoms, but I assured her it could only help. The nicotine, and what it is packaged in, is well known and documented to be toxic, as a known carcinogenic and powerfully pro-inflammatory compound. To remove that exposure would not only reduce the level of inflammation, but it might also allow her body to be more receptive to any interventions recommended by her physician, or by me. Smoking is an addiction and difficult to stop, but she worked hard to quit, and her symptoms did indeed become more tolerable and manageable once she did.

My message to her is the same one I have for you, and for me. We need to find small things we can do in our lives to either directly improve our health or increase our chance of improvement, even by small measures. It is easy to feel wooed by the idea that there is a cure for what ails us, or there is one right thing to do. But this all-or-none mentality often gets us nowhere. It is much more palatable for patients to embrace change in small steps, because then there is less of a chance of becoming discouraged or disappointed. So, for example, if you are considering dietary changes, it is much easier to start with minimization (not necessarily elimination yet) of well-known pro-inflammatory foods such as desserts and processed food. A longer-term goal can be to make bigger changes, but it's better to start small than not start at all. Similarly, movement can start with gentle stretching in your home and slowly graduate to short walks, building up from there.

Social media platforms bombard us with "fitness experts," "wellness experts," and "health experts." When faced with all these so-called experts, it is sometimes hard to be discerning, and that has nothing to do with our intelligence or education. It is just important to understand that no one has control over you and your body more than you do. You are your own best coach, support, cheerleader, and friend. I have worked with thousands of patients, and I have seen this time and time again. Those who embrace the value of their life, their being, and who they are in the world, and what they mean to those around them, are the ones who truly become their own successful advocates. You do not need a guru. You do need you. Patience with yourself, kindness to yourself, and forgiveness for yourself will help you take next steps in finding your way back to a functional baseline level of health.

Human behavior is notoriously difficult to change, and

there are many reasons for that, but breaking bad habits and developing good habits can be hard for most. "One day at a time" is a cliché, but it is true. One bad day does not make one a failure. It can give insight into what led to that bad day and how best you can avoid it again in the future.

Integrative and Effective

EVEN AS I SUGGEST TO you that you need to embrace your role as the director of your treatment journey, I also want to acknowledge the limitations and restrictions of chronic illness. You cannot move much, cannot think much, and often feel very unmotivated to make a lot of changes or even decisions that have the potential to benefit your long-term health. Maybe you have Long Covid. Maybe you have chronic fatigue syndrome. Maybe you have mast cell activation syndrome or small fiber neuropathy, or maybe you don't know what you have. You just know you have felt lousy and exhausted and racked with brain fog for who knows how long. When you feel like that, living a life of quality and joy can be hard to imagine, much less work for. The lack of motivation is likely compounded by the difficulty of finding physicians who are able to assist you in your care. Local physicians may want to help but may not feel equipped or educated on best treatment options. Physicians who do have the expertise may be too far away or no longer taking new patients, or they may be unaffordable (it is an unfortunate fact that our current insurance-directed healthcare system is untenable for physicians who need the time and autonomy to treat chronically ill patients).

As an advocate for my patients, I have seen firsthand the degree of ableism that plagues our society. Websites and social media are ablaze with directives and unsolicited advice on how to live your best life, heal your trauma, find gratitude, joy, and mindfulness. Be the person you were meant to be! All are said with good intention, I am sure. But I feel offended for my patients because their best lives, their best selves, their intentions, and their joy were taken from them and often feel out of reach. Trying to find that sense of self amid the fear that envelops them from day to day is an overwhelming burden. It makes them feel like they are at fault if they cannot find happiness in their pain and suffering. But it is not your fault. In fact, science shows us that as conscious beings we are not always in direct control of the contents of our conscious minds. So if you find you are unable to silence your mind in the midst of your fear of the loss of quality of life, it is not your fault, and you are not doing anything wrong.

Seeing patients as I have in their homes, in their beds, really drives home this point. They are often in dark, silent rooms and rely on others to help with their basic activities. Or at the least, they can no longer work their jobs, their relationships suffer, or they feel they are not able to be the parent they always dreamed they would be. They cannot do simple tasks they used to take for granted, such as going to the grocery store. There is often guilt at being a bad spouse, partner, friend, child, or parent.

I understand how lousy you may be feeling, and I know you may feel totally unmotivated and almost annoyed and just over it. And maybe you are even rolling your eyes at the things I am saying. I get it. Been there, done that. But while acknowledging these feelings, I also know that regardless of how severe your symptoms are, there are things you can do to begin to feel better or at least to feel like you are in a little bit of control. There are things you can do to try to minimize and slow progression of symptoms, and there are things you can do to try to prevent future complications of chronic disease. Again, I have worked with thousands of patients just like you, so what I say here comes from the wisdom gained from all I have done and seen. Years of practice have shown me that you can take control and feel empowered to redesign your health and life, no matter the state of your health right now. What you will find in Part II of this book is what I like to think of as one long appointment that provides you with the benefits of my experience with the many patients I have seen and taken care of over the years. The illnesses of these patients have ranged in severity—some are bedbound, and some are still working albeit part-time and usually at a slower pace—and there is a range in diagnoses from the extensive workup I do on each patient, but PEIs lend themselves to plenty of generalizations in terms of what is going on within the body both systemically and physiologically, and what effects those things have on patients' lives. My strong advice to you is to try things. Read the chapters, and embrace the things you can do today, and if you start to feel a little better, embrace more. Keep trying. Don't give up. Live a considered life—even if that consideration at this juncture is focused on your health.

My approach to treating PEIs is integrative, meaning some of the treatments require a prescription from a doctor, so while I say that you are in charge of your health, you still need a relationship with a doctor. I talk to many patients who are anti–Western medicine for various reasons, and while I am sympathetic to some of these concerns, such as the over-drugging of America and a mistrust of Big Pharma, it is important to remember that in the face of true disease and disability, pharmaceuticals can offer relief and treatment in a fast fashion and can be a lifesaver for those who need to get through a day. When I first opened my practice in 2015, I thought I would avoid using prescribed medications when able. But I soon learned the absolute benefit of prescription drugs for many symptoms my patients were experiencing. Medications have helped us recover from sickness, and Western medicine has a lot to offer, but the skill lies in knowing when to use it, how, and why. It is not useful to throw the baby out with the bathwater. The nonprescription treatments I offer are also of great benefit, with the added benefit that when nonprescription treatments are helpful, that lights the way to further treatment. You can always build on a positive response. Momentum of positive trajectory is what I aim for with my patients, whatever it may take.

Speaking of doctors, part of building that relationship involves asking questions when you have them. Importantly, if your doctor has recommended a medication, ask them about the mechanism of action of the medication (the specific way it produces an effect in the body) and why they believe it can help a particular symptom. All doctors know what the mechanism of action is for the drugs they prescribe—not only to keep you safe and to make sure you have the highest potential for benefiting from that medication, but also because knowing the mechanism of action can help them diagnose (or at least further understand) what is going in your body that is causing the symptom. If that medication does indeed offer a positive response, the mechanism of action can offer clues into what may be contributing to the symptoms and can also help the doctor decide further potential solutions. Whatever questions you have, do not leave your appointment without feeling you have gotten them answered. It is important to leave feeling satisfied, because only then can you embark on a therapeutic relationship with your doctor.

Additionally, you have the right to expect a conversation about abnormal labs from a diagnostic workup done by your doctor. Otherwise, why did they order it? Many times, patients bring me lab work or other results or tests from other providers and ask my opinion. When I ask what the ordering provider said about this abnormal finding, the patient will often shrug their shoulders. The provider either didn't say anything or dismissed it, saying it was of no significance. You may have to push a little bit to have that conversation, and for some that may be uncomfortable. But again, it is your health, and yours to be in charge of. It is all part of the work you are doing to get better and, again, it is part of the two-way relationship with your doctor.

Everything I suggest in this book I have seen work for patients. They are tried and true not only in my practice but also in the practices of other physicians I greatly respect. As progressive as I have been with my multifaceted and integrative approach in treating patients with chronic and complex illness, I am still conservative in that I have made it my business to build an arsenal of recommendations and treatments for patients in a safe and cohesive manner. I have made sure I know what to offer and when, and that my recommendations will at the very least do no harm and at the very best offer at least a small chance of improvement of symptoms and overall quality of life.

In addition to being proven effective and safe, everything I suggest in this book also is reasonable and accessible. Every suggestion holds the possibility of helping you claw your way out of the darkness of your post-viral challenge.

Be a Fighter

IT IS HARD FOR A single person to tend to themselves alone when chronically ill. It can take a village, or at least a few good friends or family members, to support you as you try for a full neurological rehab from Long Covid or another chronic and complex illness. But it starts with you, the patient. Love yourself enough to do this. I ask you to find the parts of you and your life that you are grateful for, that put a smile on your face, that make you feel even the slightest sense of joy and resilience. Trying to heal and return to a life well lived does require a certain level of dedication and commitment from you, and when you make that commitment, the support from either family or friends will follow. Many patients find powerful support from social media patient groups or from patient advocacy groups, the latter of which I think are crucial in our current healthcare environment because they help fill gaps where doctors don't have the time or inclination to guide and support patients through the morass of information (and misinformation) and directives for care associated with progressive and prolonged illnesses.

I am in this for the short haul and long haul with you. I offer ideas that have the potential of improving or minimizing symptoms now, and soon, but I also have a long game in mind. Some of the recommendations may seem cumbersome or burdensome or even impossible to take on at the moment because of your disease. But most of it is about setting the table for a future life where these recommendations are daily habits and are a new way of living. For most chronic diseases, you need a short-term and long-term plan, and I incorporate pieces of both in a very integrative manner in my practice and in this book.

You have inner strength that you have forgotten exists because you have been so burdened by your symptoms. You have spent many hours, days, weeks, months looking for a physician to listen to you, validate your symptoms, and work with you to better understand why your body and brain are functioning at a different level. The very fact you are reading this book suggests you still have hope and are willing to still fight. You have internal resilience and perseverance, even if you don't yet believe it or feel it. There is power that exists within you, and you have the autonomy to make change, however small it may be at first. It is that power that you can draw upon to give your body what it needs to heal.

Listen, I awoke from surgery unable to eat, think, dream, or believe I would ever return to some semblance of myself. I was in the dark, both literally and metaphorically. I had to claw my way back to the land of the living. And I literally could not do anything in terms of grand changes. I *had* to take small steps. My skull was being held together by staples, and pieces of my brain had just been cut out by the most barbaric of surgeries. How did I start? It was not the love of my husband or my daughter that got me there—at least not initially. It was looking at myself in the mirror and knowing I was the only one who could get this party started. And it did not require money or a large support network. It only required the belief in myself that I was not yet done.

Believe me, my doctors were not optimistic then, and to be honest, they are not optimistic now. But I decided they did not know me. Indeed, they often expressed amazement at how well I was doing. Many times, they wanted to fill out disability forms, they told me to stop working, they told me to slow down. *For what?* I would say. To sit on the couch? I have got shit to do in this lifetime, however much left there is.

I took baby steps. Then toddler steps. And so on. I needed nutrition but could not chew, so I juiced or ordered soup. I needed to move my body but could not be upright without intense headaches, so I did some stretching exercises in my bed (the yoga baby pose was my friend). I wore compression socks. I needed to sleep but couldn't because of the traumatic brain injury I had from the tumor and the surgery, so I took over-the-counter sleep medications (and some herbs). I needed to move my bowels but couldn't because bearing down caused elevated intracranial pressure, which was dangerous for me at that stage, so I took a bunch of MiraLAX (and natural stuff, which did not do the job alone!). I absolutely could not tolerate sound or light, so I stayed in a dimmed room with silence and slowly added things like meditation music that was written in specific healing frequencies for the brain (my favorite was delta wave and EMDR music). And so on. I just did what needed to be done, and all of it was cheap and on my own and did not require a single doctor, even me. But it set my path. And now here I am telling you that recovery is possible.

PART II

Strategies for Recovery

5

Nutrition, Supplements, and Medication

READ THIS CHAPTER TO FIND OUT . . .

- How to alter your diet to reduce inflammation and other chronic symptoms
- Which supplements can actually help, and which you can skip
- The role of medications in an integrative treatment approach

THE TOPICS OF DIET AND nutrition, and medication and supplements, can be bewildering. There's lots of money to be made selling diets, drugs, and "this one weird trick," which is a big reason why we see so much contradictory information shared on the internet, in books and other media, and even among friends. So you are forgiven if you have no idea where to start. What really works? What's just a fad? And your brother-in-law who eats nothing but rib eye steaks and claims to feel great—is he really okay?

Luckily, there are a few plain-and-simple guidelines for feeling better based on what you ingest. Also lucky is the fact that even small changes can help. If you're not ready to go full vegan tomorrow, or ever, you can still start feeling better with baby steps.

Avoid Foods That Stoke the Flames

PART I OF THIS BOOK has a lot to say about inflammation and how it is responsible for so many of the symptoms associated with Long Covid and other chronic conditions. Well, food can be decidedly anti-inflammatory or pro-inflammatory, and a body that has been chronically inflamed due to a PEI does not need to be stoked. Step one is to eliminate or cut way down on those foods that cause inflammation. Unfortunately, the list of inflammatory foods includes some items that can be very tempting and hard to give up: meat, dairy, processed foods, and sugar.

I often hear the argument that we need meat in our diet in order to get enough protein. This simply is not true. We do not need as much protein as we think we do, and protein, including all the necessary amino acids, can be found in non-animal foodstuffs. Some argue that meat is the only way to get vitamin B12, and while that's technically true, our bodies can hold vitamin B12 for five years,[1] which proves at the very least that we don't need to eat meat on a daily basis, and certainly not during each meal. Earlier in our evolution, we obtained our vitamin B12 from the dirt and tiny bugs on the plants that we pulled from the earth. As a neurologist, I have seen the consequences of B12 deficiency many times over the years, but significantly and quite telling, I have never seen a patient with symptomatic B12 deficiency who is a vegetarian or vegan.

Similarly, adult humans are not meant to be consuming the milk of another animal or products that are made with it. In spite of all the messaging we have heard over the decades about the supposed health benefits of dairy, it's really not good for us. Most people do not have the enzymes needed to break down parts of the dairy foods, and studies that say that dairy is good for us are usually funded by the powerful dairy lobbyists. Most important for our discussion here, dairy causes inflammation. It also increases the risk of cancer and heart disease. There are better ways to get calcium and protein.

I understand the extreme benefit and convenience of processed foods and how industrialization of food has propelled humankind, but by now I think we all also understand that the processing of foods so they have half-

---

1 Vitamin B12 Fact Sheet for Health Professionals, National Institutes of Health: Office of Dietary Supplements, updated March 26, 2024, https: //ods.od.nih.gov/factsheets/VitaminB12-HealthProfessional/.

lives longer than the lives of my dogs cannot be good for us. I'm mainly talking about ultra-processed, ready-to-eat packaged foods such as cookies, microwave meals, frozen pizzas, deli meats, chips, breakfast cereals, and so on. They are hard to avoid, and hard to resist! Not only are these foods convenient, but most people find them to be delicious. Of course, the reason they're so delicious is because they're loaded with sodium and sugar, two big culprits of inflammation. They also tend to be loaded with cholesterol-spiking trans fats and potentially cancer-causing preservatives.

We know sugar is addicting, and studies have shown that the physiologic effects of consuming sugar are similar to using illicit drugs. The more we eat, the more we want. Too much sugar over time causes a continual release of insulin, meant to remove glucose from the bloodstream and help the cells take it in, but eventually our bodies can no longer manage the level of sugar in the blood, and sugar molecules attach themselves to our cells and become a burden to their functioning. Many people are aware that sugar feeds cancer cells, but less well known is the fact that it also feeds other atypical cells. Sugar glycosylation—the attachment of sugar components to cellular tissues—makes it harder for cells to do their jobs. Processed sugars are useless to our mitochondria, the organelles in our cells that produce energy, and they clog up the machinery so that real substrates that make energy do not have access. When the mitochondria cannot work as they should, energy supply is less available, and cells that *really* need energy, such as the very active brain, do not get it and cannot work, which results in sluggish thinking and poor mental clarity, or brain fog. Sugar also, of course, contributes to systemic and neural inflammation. There are a multitude of reasons, with robust science behind them, for why sugar should be at the very least minimized but preferably avoided.

The medical and scientific evidence in favor of a plant-based diet is overwhelming.[2] While I have been plant-based and vegan for several decades, I recognize that such a diet is not ideal for everyone, nor is it easy. I don't preach or condemn, and it's not my goal to make everyone into a vegan, though I think we can all agree that we, and our planet, would all do well if we included more plant-based foods in our diet. I also believe some patients when they tell me they feel better when they eat animal meat. Human metabolism is complex and genetically based, and the variations among us are based on ancestry, environment, and state of health or disease, so there are likely real reasons behind why some patients do well with a little animal meat in their diets.

Nevertheless, cutting down on unhealthy food choices, many of which may be habitual or even cultural, can help. Here's where those baby steps come in. If you eat meat

---

2 Angelo Capodici et al., "Cardiovascular Health and Cancer Risk Associated with Plant Based Diets: An Umbrella Review," *PLoS ONE* 19, no. 5: https://doi.org/10.1371/journal.pone.0300711; Elaine Hillesheim et al., "Association of Plant-Based Diet Indexes with the Metabolomic Profile," *Scientific Reports* 14 (August 2024): https://doi.org/10.1038/s41598-024-68522-4.

seven days a week, start by cutting down to five at first. If you consume lots of dairy, perhaps you can reduce it by going to black coffee instead of mixing in cream, or trying a plant-based creamer—they have gotten quite tasty. And so on. Each day we have at least one chance, though usually more, to choose foods that will not stoke the fire of inflammation but will instead help to calm it. It really is that simple. And the best part is that even when we make a poor choice, we have the chance to make a better choice at our next meal.

There is one other category of foods to avoid, a category that is much harder to define: foods you are intolerant to. I don't mean foods you are allergic to, which of course you should avoid. But mast cells are of high concentration along the lining of the gastrointestinal tract, and if they are reactive, then the mere presence of foodstuffs in the stomach and in the intestine can further their reactivity and hence create lots of inflammation. The work that is required to digest, absorb, and use the macro- and micronutrients of the foods we eat is that much harder. Many patients develop a very limited repertoire of foods that they are able to tolerate. This leads to not only nutritional deficiencies but also an unhealthy microbiome, which is the collection of species that live in our tract. An unhealthy microbiome has unhealthy communication with the central and peripheral nervous systems.

It is important to try to understand which foods you tolerate and which ones you don't tolerate as well. This may take some detective work, and a nutritionist can be a great resource to help you navigate elimination diets or specialized diets such as low-FODMAP (fermentable oligosaccharides, disaccharides, monosaccharides, and polyols). Pay close attention to how your body feels after eating, especially when it does not feel good. Do you develop nausea, heartburn, or diarrhea? Take note of what you ate. Other symptoms to look for include a change of urinary or bowel habits, muscle fatigue, cognitive fatigue, or headache. If you're having reactions like these, it can help to keep a food journal. For several weeks, record exactly what you eat for every meal and how your body reacts. You should be able to discern some patterns after a while. Once you identify a food or foods that may be causing an adverse reaction, give that food up for a while and see if the symptoms go away. It may take some time and, as I say, some detective work, but it can be worth it.

But just as important is to work to reduce the activity of those inflammatory pesky cells that are making it an inhospitable environment even for foods you previously enjoyed without any problems. Reducing the activity of the mast cells but also reducing the level of inflammation can be key to improving the health of your gut. Antihistamines that are over the counter are helpful, as are some supplements such as quercetin. There are many medications that your doctor can prescribe. Some important herbal formulations are licorice tincture, marshmallow tincture, and ginger.

The Ketogenic Diet: Yea or Nay?

MANY OF MY PATIENTS ASK me if they should try the ketogenic ("keto") diet. It has become quite popular with people trying to lose weight, gain mental clarity, and alleviate other health concerns, with many internet personalities (and perhaps people in your own life) proclaiming how it has changed their life. My short answer for those patients who are interested in trying it, and for you, if you're interested, is that it may be helpful if you want to try it for a short time. My patients who know I am vegan always give me the side-eye when I tell them to go for it, like, *What do you* really *think?* What I really think is that it can be helpful for a while, but the key to remember is that it is not a long-term solution.

A ketogenic diet simply means eliminating carbohydrates and getting your calories exclusively, or almost exclusively, from fat and protein—foods like meat, fish, eggs, and nuts. When you eliminate carbs, especially fast-digesting carbs like sugary desserts, soda, white bread, and so on, you eliminate glucose as an energy source, and eventually your body will turn to protein and fat for energy. And it gets very good at using fat, which is why people lose weight. When you're in this state where your body is burning protein and fat for energy, you're in ketosis.

Besides weight loss, there are other benefits to being in ketosis, most importantly reducing or eliminating seizures in patients who don't respond to any of the many anti-seizure drugs available today.[3] The brain's preferred fuel is glucose, and for patients who have a very sensitive brain—and who don't respond to any other treatment—even a little glucose can set off a seizure. If medications do not work to manage the seizures, we may introduce the ketogenic diet in order to remove the glucose molecule. When we take away the molecule that it loves so much, we hope that it no longer uses that fuel to seize. It works in about 50 percent of patients. And when it works, it really is amazing. I have seen patients go from having multiple seizures a day to none, just from being in ketosis.

Being in ketosis can also be a huge relief for patients suffering from lots of inflammation due to a PEI. This diet offers some absolutely healthy benefits in the short term, and it can really help alleviate that inflammation. You may experience a bump in energy initially, as well as less pain, less brain fog, all from taking away the glucose. If you have been sick for a long time, if you have been experiencing lots of inflammation, then you have a sensitive brain just like those patients who have chronic seizures, but you also have a sensitive gut and other sensitive systems. Getting rid of the glucose gives your body a break. The glucose has been stoking the fire for so long, you have been inflamed for so long, your body needs a rest. I estimate that 80 percent of

---

3 Cristina Díez-Arroyo et al., "Effect of the Ketogenic Diet as a Treatment for Refractory Epilepsy in Children and Adolescents: A Systematic Review of Reviews," *Nutrition Reviews* 82, no. 4 (April 2024): 487–502, https://doi.org/10.1093/nutrit/nuad071.

the patients I start on a keto diet come back in four weeks and say they feel better. They're thinking better, sleeping better, they have more energy. But here's the thing: The majority of them come back in six months and are no longer feeling better.

The reason for that is that the brain prefers the glucose molecule for its fuel. The brain will be happy for a while to use the fatty acids, but it takes too much energy to use fatty acids for energy for brain function, and after a while the brain gets tired and starts to rebel. You're basically starving the brain of what it needs. After a few months on a keto diet, you will find that you can't think straight, you are incredibly fatigued, you have brain fog. All those symptoms you were trying to get rid of? They're back.

And you may have other side effects from doing a ketogenic diet long term. People, even young people, may develop cardiovascular disease, cerebrovascular disease, kidney stones, or cognitive difficulties. On top of that, eating all that fat is not good for your other organs, including the GI tract. It's hard for your body to metabolize a lot of fat, and studies show that metabolites of animal protein foods can be toxic to the body. The more you eat, the more they accumulate in the blood and can become toxic.

I do support my patients who want to try a ketogenic diet, but I'm very clear with them that it should be a short-term solution. Get your body into ketosis, then give it a break. And we need to work toward other solutions. And in fact, there is a better way to get the body into ketosis, one that is much easier to stick to long term, and one that has only positive health benefits: intermittent fasting.

The Benefits of Intermittent Fasting

A FEW YEARS AGO, A couple came to see me because they were both suffering from chronic headaches, low energy, difficulty breathing, dizziness, rashes, joint pain, and more. The symptoms had started years earlier, and they'd been seeing various doctors to no avail. Then one day they found black mold growing in their bathroom and, assuming this was the culprit, they had it remediated. Walls were torn down, experts brought in, the whole home was cleaned out. But getting rid of the mold did not help. They continued seeing doctors, they read every book they could find about mold exposure and how to recover, but still: those headaches, that fatigue, the breathing challenges, and the rest. The woman, Paula, had epilepsy, which she was treating effectively with medication, but she was worried that these continued symptoms might make it worse. She was an opera singer, and even her voice had suffered. Roberto, the husband, had diabetes and cardiovascular disease, and he too was worried about his conditions getting worse. She was in her late forties, and he was in his early fifties.

By the time Paula and Roberto came to me, it had been two years since they'd had the house remediated. They had tried mold exposure treatment and been to doctors who are "mold experts," and they had tried several different medications, but they were still sick. They still had this post-exposure illness. I did my usual workup on them, which included a bunch of labs and MRIs, and which showed a lot of inflammation. No medications had worked to cure them, so I focused on alleviating symptoms. We looked at their lifestyle. She was a singer and he was a lawyer, so they both had stressful jobs that involved a lot of travel. We looked at their sleep schedule, which was messed up due to the traveling. But mainly we looked at diet.

They both ate a typical American diet. Meat, dairy, occasional desserts. Because they traveled so much, they often found themselves eating at restaurants on the fly—a sandwich and fries, a burger and chips, deep-fried anything. And I told them, I get it. You're on the road, you're looking for what's convenient. But when you're sick, convenience does not matter as much. If you eat like that, you're going to get sicker. I told them what I tell all my patients: Food is medicine. They were willing to make changes but wondered what their options were, and I suggested that they not eat when they're traveling.

"What?" they asked. "Don't eat? Like, anything?"

They were taking these long trips where they were in airplanes and airports for twelve hours. I said, "Just don't eat during that time. Give your body a break. Just fast," I said. "You'll live."

This is something I recommend all the time. It's also something that, like the ketogenic diet, is trendy these days and all over the internet. But unlike the keto diet, I recommend intermittent fasting with no reservations. For one thing, you can get the benefits of the keto diet—which is a state of ketosis, or no glucose in the system—but you're not ingesting huge amounts of hard-to-digest fat, and you're not depriving your brain of its preferred fuel for months at a time. And you can get a wide range of nutrients.

Intermittent fasting is a beneficial behavior for a multitude of reasons, including, to begin, giving your body that break and therefore reducing inflammation. It helps protect our mitochondria. It protects our nerve cells against damage or degeneration, and it is generally good for our overall longevity.[4] When we are in a fasted state, blood is diverted from the gastrointestinal tract to other organs, and that can boost blood supply to the brain, heart, lungs, muscles, and more. When we eat, blood rushes to the gastrointestinal tract to help with digestion, metabolism, and absorption. That often makes us feel fatigued and sluggish because blood supply elsewhere is poor. This is exacerbated in the chronically ill population because of

---

4 Daniele Lettieri-Barbato et al., "Time-Controlled Fasting Prevents Aging-Like Mitochondrial Changes Induced by Persistent Dietary Fat Overload in Skeletal Muscle," *PLoS ONE* (May 2018): https://doi.org/10 .1371/journal.pone.0195912; Yihang Zhao, Mengzhen Jia, Weixuan Chen, and Zhigang Liu, "The Neuroprotective Effects of Intermittent Fasting on Brain Aging and Neurodegenerative Diseases via Regulating Mitochondrial Function," *Free Radical Biology and Medicine* 182 (2022): 206–18, https://doi.org/10.1016/j.freeradbiomed.2022.02.021.

the extent of connective tissue degeneration, and because the blood vessels are not as strong as they need to be to hold and support the passage of blood. The inflammatory barriers along the vessel walls slow down the necessary perfusion of the blood. Intermittent fasting has been shown to boost cognition; improve focus, attention, and concentration; improve energy supply to muscles; increase overall energy; deepen our sleep; and enhance digestive functions. There is robust research proving the health benefits of intermittent fasting for everyone, even for those who are not chronically sick. We Americans eat too much. You take a two-and-a-half-hour plane flight, and they come down the aisle offering snacks. We can make it two and a half hours without eating! We are not letting our organs rest, ever. We are constantly eating, metabolizing, and digesting, and this causes a lot of imbalance in the gut microbiome. Intermittent fasting allows blood to be diverted to the brain and other places besides the gut.

There are a few different ways to do intermittent fasting, including having a normal diet for some days and completely fasting on other days, but that is not what I'm talking about here. I recommend daily, time-restricted fasting in which you eat every day but only within a certain period of time. It's commonly recommended that you limit eating to an eight-hour window, and that is great, but the timing of those hours is more important than the number of hours. It is best to simulate our natural circadian rhythms. So, while it may be easier for many to hold off on breakfast in the morning, it is more effective and more therapeutic to fast later in the day and eat a small, early dinner.

We have developed social norms over decades that may be fun and engaging, such as eating a late dinner and especially going out to dinner late at night, but these habits are not good for our long-term health. Going out to eat usually means pro-inflammatory foods and alcohol, and eating late in general usually means going to bed with undigested food in our stomachs or somewhere along our tracts.

Instead, have a small meal around five P.M. and don't eat any more that evening, with a plan of going to bed without food in your stomach and maybe even with a slight feeling of hunger. This will improve your sleep and help you feel more refreshed the next morning. Your sleep will be better consolidated, which not only ensures optimal glymphatic function—the process of clearing away waste in the brain, including irritating substances—but also helps to cement lessons learned from memories made earlier that day.[5] Memory and learning take place during the night after the lessons of the day. If you learn something during the day, a good, healthy, restorative night of sleep will help make sure you have gotten the most out of that new information—be it at school, at work, with

---

5 K. I. Voumvourakis et al., "The Dynamic Relationship Between the Glymphatic System, Aging, Memory, and Sleep," *Biomedicines* 11, no. 8 (2023): 2092, https://doi.org/10.3390/biomedicines11082092.

friends, with family, or even just leisure reading. There are so many health rewards from improved sleep that we will discuss further in Chapter 8, but one piece is to simulate the rhythm of sleep and wakefulness. Intermittent fasting in this fashion can play a role. I promise you will feel better in the morning after sleeping without foodstuffs that need to be attended to in your body. Another important note is the activity of the microbiome is different during the day than it is at night, and the consequences of an altered microbiome are worse when the bacterium get to feed at night.

As a side note, I mentioned alcohol previously, and I want to point out that alcohol causes laxity of tissues, and when we lie in bed after even one or two drinks, there is too much laxity of everything from the esophagus to the lower colon, and stuff we ate is more likely to sit stagnant. Not to mention the effects on our trachea, also made of connective tissue, which is why many will snore when they drink, and most will have non-restorative sleep with frequent awakenings after a night of even a few drinks. There is also commonly GI upset with gas, diarrhea, and discomfort. Even under the best conditions, I do not believe any amount of alcohol is healthy. But especially for my chronically ill patients who are suffering the constant assault of an immune and inflammatory response, I recommend no alcohol.

So, how to begin with intermittent fasting? Again, you can start with baby steps. Have your breakfast a little later than usual, maybe an hour later just to extend the fast by an hour or two. It's okay to have a cup of tea or black coffee but skip the cream and sugar. Can you eat dinner a little earlier, too? Try not to eat or drink anything after dinner. Give your body several hours to digest before going to bed. Try to get your window of eating down to ten hours, then later go to nine.

The choice of foods you eat is another critical component. Pro-inflammatory foods are a burden to the enzymatic fires of our body that no amount of intermittent fasting can easily counteract. You already know what to avoid: dairy, processed foods, sugar. To achieve best results, target dark leafy greens, legumes, grains, cruciferous vegetables, and root vegetables, which are full of phytonutrients—chemicals produced by plants that are antioxidant and anti-inflammatory, and that are necessary for the thousands of biochemical reactions that happen in our body every day. They're also loaded with vitamins that feed the enzymes that do this heavy work for us.

In the end, it's all about using your common sense. Intermittent fasting is more about the timing of your diet than the substance of it. It's all about giving your gut a break. But it's best to avoid inflammatory foods, too, right? What is the point of trying to reduce and avoid inflammation if you eat fast food each day? Do your best and build from there. Once you start seeing results, it will feel a lot easier to make bigger changes.

The Benefits of Juicing

PAULA AND ROBERTO, THE COUPLE with the mold exposure, embraced intermittent fasting and the whole idea of improving their diets, and within a few months they were feeling a lot better. They were no longer eating meat, they ate more salads, and they were choosing dark leafy greens over iceberg lettuce. They were fasting more and more because they traveled so much, and they didn't eat while in airports or airplanes. They felt less fatigue, had fewer headaches, and had more clarity in their thinking. None of this happened overnight. It was small changes. One good meal choice followed by another. When we added juicing to the mix, things really took off. They began by juicing a few meals a week, and eventually they were juicing their breakfast every day. Before long, the improvements they'd already experienced got even better—clear head, no headaches, no joint pain, no fatigue. In fact, they had more energy than they could ever remember having. Paula's voice improved, and so did her performances. Even more remarkable was what happened to Roberto. His diabetes improved to the point where he could reduce his insulin intake. He'd been diabetic since his twenties, and this was the first time he was able to reduce insulin requirements. Not only that—he lost forty pounds.

The power of food as medicine is not just a catchphrase or a hashtag, and it really cannot be denied. Evolution has made it so we perceive sugar and oil as tasty because long ago they were in short supply (plant foods do not contain either). Entities that sell such foods take advantage of this primitive urge, which is based deep in the limbic system. But these foods are no longer in short supply. They are everywhere—every restaurant, café, drive-through, market, and gas station. Sugar and grease are cheap and easy to buy and cheap and easy to eat. For a brief moment during and after eating them, you may feel a sense of elation, euphoria, even satisfaction. But that emotion is fleeting, and then your body takes on the consequence of the inflammatory assault.

On the other hand, when we eat whole foods—foods that are natural and not processed—and focus on a wide variety of colorful fruits and vegetables, we feel great because those foods are loaded with the phytonutrients that are so good for us. A great way to do that is through juicing, which I recommend to all my patients, and which I recommend to you, and which I personally do every day. It's a great way to reduce inflammation and get tons of phytonutrients fast. While I cannot eat three bunches of kale, I can juice them. While I cannot eat four apples in one sitting, I can juice them. I make a green juice each morning and an apple juice each afternoon. It helps me to absorb increased quantities of vitamins and minerals without relying too much on supplementation and is a great way to start my day.

Juicing is easy on an inflamed gastrointestinal tract

and helps hydrate us, an important factor for patients with chronic illness. Drinking free water does not improve hydration as much as we would like to think it does since healthy, functioning kidneys will excrete free water. The kidneys are designed to sense balance between osmoles (ions) in the plasma and water, and when they're not in balance, the kidneys will excrete either the water or the osmoles, mainly the sodium ions. That is why it is recommended that patients either take salt tabs with their water or add electrolyte powders to their water bottles, as athletes do. Many vegetables, such as cucumbers, and fruits, such as watermelon, contain natural electrolytes and sodium and also have high water content. Juicing can accomplish so much in the efforts to heal.

Juicing removes the fiber, so it is a concentrated source of phytonutrients that our bodies need to function and to heal. Fiber is good for the motility of the GI tract as well as for the health of the microbiome (those bugs that hang out in your gut), so you should definitely eat whole fruits and whole vegetables—but you won't be able to eat too much in one sitting *because* of the bulk. Smoothies, on the other hand, are pulverized fruits and vegetables with all the fiber, and that is often very hard for many of my patients because it is like an "osmotic load," meaning the bulk creates an environment within the GI tract that does not feel good. It can cause distension, gas, nausea, diarrhea, and, just as important, make the mast cells upset along with the residents of the microbiome.

Juicing to Help Handle Chemical Exposure

Every six months I get an MRI with gadolinium, a chemical that is administered intravenously in order to provide contrast for the imaging. To say I am *not* happy with this level of exposure would be an understatement. But I understand why the contrast is needed. To prepare for my exposure, I fast the day before and the morning of. After the MRI, I drink a freshly made juice of red and yellow beets, parsley, apple, pineapple, turmeric root, and ginger, with ten drops of gromwell and ashwagandha. I drink the same juice the next day as well. I always do fine with the MRI and have no aftereffects from the exposure.

Part of the juicing conversation I have with patients usually focuses on some of the perceived obstacles, starting with purchasing a juicer. They can be quite expensive, but there are affordable models, and I definitely recommend starting with one of the cheaper options. If the cost of buying large amounts of fresh fruits and vegetables is a barrier, you can mix in frozen versions, which are just as healthy but more affordable. The shopping, prep, and cleanup are other obstacles. And I get it. Look, I go to the store four or five times a week. It's a pain in the ass. But I'm telling you it's worth it. My advice is to jump in and give it a try. We have talked about baby steps, but even baby steps start with step one, then step two, and so on. Try to be consistent so that you get used to the process and it feels less new and less arduous. Over time, with consistency, juicing becomes a habit, and the prep, process, and cleanup is just part of your morning routine. As you begin to appreciate the benefits—from reduced inflammation and pain to clearer focus and higher energy—you may become invested in the process.

That's what happened with Paula and Roberto. They had removed the mold, which was the exposure that had triggered their chronic conditions, but by then they were already hypersensitive to all sorts of exposures, and they had not removed everything else that was inflaming their bodies. Someone who does not have a PEI can eat an inflammatory meal, and it's okay. They might not feel that great, but their body will get over it. Eventually they will feel fine again. But for Paula and Roberto, and for anyone else with a PEI, after that initial damaging exposure, any small exposure was too much. Their bodies no longer had any resilience. The solution was to take what was further inflaming their bodies and remove it. They were not 100 percent better in six months, but they were 60 to 70 percent better.

Sprouting

I also highly recommend sprouting—growing sprouts from seeds or beans—which is surprisingly easy to do at home with very inexpensive equipment (jars) and seeds (you can buy six months' worth of seeds for mere dollars). The sprouts of seeds and legumes contain highly

concentrated forms of protein and have a dense nutritional value of unique quality. For example, broccoli
sprouts are a very potent source of sulforaphane, an important compound for brain health as it helps to reduce
neuroinflammation and eats up free radicals, which can
be toxic to the brain cells. And sprouts are delicious. I
add them to soup, salad, and sandwiches.

What's even better about juicing is that different recipes containing different specific fruits or vegetables can target different symptoms and concerns. You can tailor your juices to your specific needs in the same way you might tailor your use of supplements and other treatments. Here are some rough guidelines to get you started:

TO HELP WITH THIS	MIX THIS INTO YOUR JUICE
Brain Fog	Turmeric and Ginger
Headaches	Cucumber
Bloating	Celery
Rash	Apples
Fatigue	Yellow or Red Beets

Here are a few of my favorite juicing recipes.

APPLE JUICE

I like to make this in the afternoon to help deal with midday fatigue and lapsing motivation (instead of coffee!).

Turmeric: 3-inch piece of root
Black pepper: ¼ teaspoon
Garlic: 5 cloves
Apples: 3 whole
Sometimes I add radishes (3 of them)

GREEN JUICE

This is my usual morning green juice, and there is no better way to get the day started. These ingredients are full of phytonutrients for energy production by the cells and a start of the engines for the organs, as well as the perfect nutritional boost a body needs after fasting during sleep.

Cucumbers: 2 whole
Kale: 1 bunch
Parsley: 1 bunch
Turmeric: 2-inch piece of root
Ginger: 1 inch

Lemon: 1 whole peeled
Sunchoke: 1 medium

Side note about turmeric: If possible, buy real turmeric root and juice it. I don't think any brand that capsulizes turmeric is worth its weight in salt. Ground spice form is okay, but in supplement form it is not bioavailable.

MAST CELL ACTIVATION JUICE

Here is my juice recipe for mast cell activation symptoms. I will occasionally drink this in the morning instead of my usual green juice. These ingredients are natural sources of quercetin, a plant pigment that helps to stabilize mast cells and has antihistamine and anticoagulant properties. This juice will also help move your bowels.

Apples: 4 whole
Red grapes: 4 bunches
Pears: 2 whole (any variety)
Parsley: ½ bunch
Ionic minerals: 2 dropperfuls

Supplements

WHEN I OPENED MY PRIVATE practice back in 2015, I had already done a lot of work in integrative medicine, which is a practice of medicine that combines conventional and mainstream approaches with alternative and Eastern approaches; the combination is tailored for the individual patient, and was decidedly dedicated to the idea of trying hard to avoid the use of medications for patients. The plan, as I envisioned it, was to first consider supplements and other alternative treatments to treat patients, and for a while that is what I did. But it was a very different practice when I first opened. I often laugh at how much time I had to eat my lunch and go for a midday walk back in the early days. Those days are over, and I am proud of the work I have done to help patients since I entered this space of chronic and complex illness. As I began working with this patient population, patients who had been battling myriad symptoms related to immune system overload for months and years, it quickly became clear that supplements were not going to help them. In a short amount of time, I developed a different perspective on the utility and use of supplements. I hope you will hear me on this because it is coming from an integrative doctor who was a true believer in the power of supplements: Supplements, especially in the oral form, are not going to be a curative solution for you while you are chronically ill. They may play an ancillary or supportive role, but they are not going to offer significant or sustained response to get you to where I want you to be.

I do believe that nutraceuticals, the commonly used term to describe supplements and other alternative medicinal food products, have a role in the care of chronic illness, particularly in prevention and even in maintenance once the patient is doing better. But that role, which should definitely be *supplemental*, has gotten cloudy for many because the world of supplements has gotten out of hand. There is a manufactured pill for just about every vitamin or mineral that can be found in nature and in our bodies. And there are formulations for just about everything that ails us—gut health, mitochondrial health, brain health, nerve health, anxiety, sleep, and more. New brands are constantly popping up as many doctors try to get in the supplement game and put their name on something. Supplements are completely unregulated, which means you can also buy them at any corner store, and studies have shown that many brands don't contain more than a trace of the actual vitamin or nutrient or mineral they claim to have. It's like the Wild West. Patients often come into my clinic with a bag of pill bottles, and most of them they don't even know why they were told to take them or even if they are helping. How could they know, when they are taking so many? The idea that anyone should be on twenty different supplements just seems foolish to me.

And, as we work to avoid processed foods, it seems a harsh contradiction to consume processed vitamins. They are not simply available in nature waiting to be packaged for supplemental consumption. Each must first be formulated to make it bioavailable so it even has a chance of efficacy, and also to make it stable, safe, and tolerable, which can be a challenge. Excipients (inactive substances) are added to help keep the product stable, and then it is manufactured in either tablet form or put into a plastic capsule—all highly processed. And excipients and the added plastic can be the enemy of those who already suffer with mast cell sensitivity and reactivity, because they just add fuel to a fire that is already threatening to be unwieldy. It is hard for our natural enzymes and immune barriers to recognize the vitamin or mineral in a tablet or capsule form. Finally, there are no studies that prove the safety of the use of multiple supplements, and they could conceivably have interactions with one another. For these reasons, even when I do recommend supplements, usually as part of a personalized and tailored plan for patients, I generally do not recommend them in the forms of capsules or tablets and very much prefer those in tincture, liquid, or powdered form because they are less processed and decidedly more bioavailable.

My even stronger recommendation, as you know by now, is to find whole food sources for these supplements, as many, though unfortunately not all, exist in nature to some extent. I try to fulfill patients' needs for most nutrients through their nutrition plan. For one thing, our bodies work best when fueled by the wide balance of nutrients that comes from natural foods. Phytonutrients in fruits and veggies provide a balanced mix of vitamins, minerals, and antioxidants. And those nutrients work together to help one another get absorbed in the body and do their jobs better. As an added bonus, fruits and veggies come with lots of fiber, which is great for your digestion. Supplements usually don't have fiber. Besides all that, eating good food is just nicer. Many people get nausea and stomach upset from swallowing supplements, and they have to spend time scheduling when they will take what. Why would we choose to swallow plastic capsules several times a day when we could obtain our necessary vitamins for functioning within a delicious meal?

Having said all the above, I will recommend a select few supplements. When I work with my patients and can get to know them and their condition, I will tailor recommendations for each patient to target their most prominent symptoms and concerns. Assuming there is no identified deficiency, which is a practical reason for supplementation, I usually suggest some combination of the following to most patients for support of healing from chronic illness:

- Magnesium
- Quercetin
- Boswellia
- Ashwagandha
- Palmitoylethanolamide (PEA)
- Coenzyme Q10

These six supplements are crucial for much of what our bodies are put through. Magnesium, which comes in many different salts (I prefer glycinate or threonate), is an important element for several enzymes and helps to stabilize vessel walls to support blood flow.[6] Quercetin helps to stabilize mast cells and has antihistamine and anticoagulant properties.[7] Boswellia has been shown to reduce cerebral edema and neuroinflammation.[8] Ashwagandha is an incredible adaptogen that modulates the body's response to stress and helps to relax our neuroendocrine axis and sympathetic drive.[9] Palmitoylethanolamide is an autacoid that is anti-inflammatory.[10] Coenzyme Q10 helps to boost the mitochondria so that the inflammatory response is less chaotic and more controlled.[11]

---

6 A. C. Montezano, T. T. Antunes, G. Callera, and R. M. Touyz, "Magnesium and Vessels," in *Encyclopedia of Metalloproteins*, eds. R. H. Kretsinger et al. (New York: Springer, 2013), https://doi.org/10.1007/978-1-4614-1533-6_267.

7 Ay Muhammet et al., "Quercetin," in *Nutraceuticals*, ed. Ramesh C. Gupta (Academic Press, 2016): 447–52, https://doi.org/10.1016/B978-0-12-802147-7.00032-2.

8 Ronald E. Warnick, "Treatment of Adverse Radiation Effects with *Boswellia serrata* After Failure of Pentoxifylline and Vitamin E: Illustrative Cases," *Journal of Neurosurgery* 5, no. 5 (January 2023): https://doi.org/10.3171/CASE22488.

9 Sultan Zahiruddin et al., "Ashwagandha in Brain Disorders: A Review of Recent Developments," *Journal of Ethnopharmacology* 257, no. 112876 (July 2020): https://doi.org/10.1016/j.jep.2020.112876.

10 Paul Clayton et al., "Palmitoylethanolamide: A Natural Compound for Health Management," *International Journal of Molecular Sciences* 22, no. 10 (May 2021): 5305, https://www.ncbi.nlm.nih.gov/pmc/articles/PMC8157570/.

11 Catarina M. Quinzii and Michio Hirano, "Coenzyme Q and Mitochondrial Disease," *Developmental Disabilities Research Reviews* 16, no. 2 (June 2010): 183–88, https://www.ncbi.nlm.nih.gov/pmc/articles/PMC3097389/.

There are others I will recommend, of course, along the path of recovery with patients. Unfortunately, I cannot sit with each of you to figure out your best course of action with regard to supplements, so what I recommend instead is that you work with your own doctor before starting or continuing any supplements.

When You Talk to Your Doctor About . . .
Supplements

Ideally, you have a doctor whom you trust and have a strong therapeutic relationship with. If they suggest a supplement, ask them which brand they recommend and why. Ask them if the supplement is available in tincture, liquid, or powdered form, and if they recommend capsule form, ask them if they are aware of any studies that confirm the amount of the compound in the capsule as opposed to excipients. Also ask if there are any side effects you should be concerned with and if there are interactions with other supplements you may be taking, or your medications.

Also discuss the plan with regard to how long to try the supplement, when and if to increase dosage, what improvements you are looking for that can be attributed to the supplement, and at what point you and your doctor will decide the supplement is not helping and you should discontinue it.

If you start a supplement, or if you have been on one for any length of time, it's important to be honest with yourself. Keep in mind the specific symptom that the supplement is supposed to address, and ask yourself if it is improving. Do you feel better? Or do you just wish you did? These are paid for completely out of pocket, and many of them can be quite costly, so be as objective as you can in assessing that, and if it's not helping you, then stop taking it.

I want to specifically address multivitamins, which are a waste of money. They contain a little of everything and not enough of anything, and you lose most of what is there when you pee. If you are eating an even moderately varied diet, you are likely getting the bare minimum of the necessary concentration for these vitamins. The same applies to formulations of things that are named after the symptom or disorder they are purporting to treat. While I understand that these "cocktails" of several different supplements save a lot of time and money, they are just not as effective as individual supplements that are known to be of high quality and are of direct benefit for what you are trying to treat or overcome. When it comes to supplements, targeted use of high-quality brands is really the only cost-effective way to go.

There's no doubt: Regularly maintaining healthy meals on a daily basis is a lot of work, and without support it may be a large obstacle for many who are unable to shop, prep, and cook. It also may be difficult to eat enough of these foods, which by their nature are dense and fibrous, for a body that is under-functioning and is rife with mast cell activity, autoimmunity, connective tissue failure, and fatigue. Under these circumstances, supplements are a way of obtaining nutrients, because recovery to any extent is even harder without a good nutritional status. If a vitamin deficiency has been clearly identified, and certainly if the symptoms correlate with the known effects of that vitamin deficiency, supplementation is the only answer. But again, I recommend the liquid or tincture formulations of supplements because they are more bioavailable and less toxic. I also prefer the new forms of alternative vitamins available such as food bites or powders that you can mix with water—or your juice.

Medications

I SEE MANY PATIENTS WHO prefer to avoid medications and to treat their symptoms as naturally as possible, and I for sure will help them do that when it's appropriate. But it's not always appropriate. When we do not feel well, and have not felt well for a long time, natural approaches often do not work fast enough to provide us with relief. Besides that, they require consistency and compliance in order to have a benefit at all, and for those who have been chronically ill, time and patience are often in short supply. The same applies to dietary interventions, by the way. When we are short on reserves of energy, motivation, and commitment, we will not only crave more comfort foods, but we will not be able to make the effort necessary to buy, prepare, cook, eat, and clean up after more nutritionally dense meals.

Medications, on the other hand, are designed to work fast. And medications can sometimes help doctors tailor a more personalized natural approach in other areas, because a patient's response to a particular medication provides insight and perspective into what's wrong with them. If a patient responds well to a medication, then we know better what we are targeting. Having more objective data on what your body responds to can be useful for recommendations of other treatment and management options.

Medications don't come without their own risk of side effects, of course, and a risk of overt toxicity. Anyone can be allergic to anything, so if you take a dose of a prescribed medication and have an adverse effect or symptom, let your doctor know right away so they can discontinue that medication and move on to something else in terms of treatment. That is the nature of complex disease. Side effects are the norm and often pose an obstacle for many mast cell activation patients, whether they are due to the medicinal compound itself or the excipients. To sort this out, it is important to ask your doctor to help you get your medication compounded so it can be made without the excipients. Compounding is the process of mixing a customized version of a drug so the ingredients can be precisely tailored to the individual patient, and as part of that you can have excipients excluded or minimized. That is not possible for all medications, but it is possible for most. It's also possible for some supplements. It is definitely worth a try, because it can be so easy to presume a medication "failed" or that you did not "tolerate" medication when that is not really known until the medication or the supplement is tried without the excipient, filler, or preservative with which it is packaged.

When You Talk to Your Doctor About . . .
Compounding a Medication

If you have been suffering from the chronic conditions described in this book, I recommend that any medications you take be compounded if that is possible (not all medications can be compounded). If your prescribing doctor does not suggest it during your visit, don't hesitate to bring it up yourself: "I'm worried that excipient ingredients in the medication can make some symptoms worse. What are my options for getting a compounded version?" Very few doctors can compound on site, but there are many compounding pharmacies throughout the country. Some are even mail order, so they can ship to wherever you may live. It may be helpful to have a conversation with the pharmacist and ask what the excipients and fillers are in the medication in question and what the risk of sensitivities are to those excipients and fillers.

Unfortunately, the cost of compounded medication is usually higher than it is for non-compounded medication, and insurance may not cover it, but if you can afford it, the difference is worthwhile.

Sometimes patients with chronic illness can tolerate small dosing of medications even if they are not compounded if they are also treated with mast cell stabilizers, antihistamines, and other medications that counteract some of the side effects caused by excipients. Many of my patients are so familiar with their body's response to various medications, supplements, and even foods that they are very adept at managing it on their own and will often take a much smaller dose than what I have recommended. You may very well have similar familiarity with your body's response to medications, and though I encourage you to take precautions that you know you need to take, please be in close contact with your doctor before altering your dosage or quitting a medication.

Some disease is caused or flared by an individual's response to a medication. If it is a commonly used medication, many doctors won't necessarily believe it—that a short course of a very common medication could have wreaked such havoc in an individual body even though they have prescribed it so many times. Or maybe the patients themselves have taken the medication before and tolerated it well but now are feeling diffuse symptoms that do not seem to get better. This is similar to a cumulative exposure. Exposure could be to anything external and does not have to always be an infection. I have many patients who became ill after a course of certain medications. Deep dives into the mechanism by which those medications work and then into that patient's unique genes and their variants often give me at least a clue of what may be happening with the patient. Again, find doctors who are not only caring but curious.

Bottom line, as an integrative neurologist, I do very much advocate for medications when we need to treat something now or fast or something severe and progressive. Why should you continue to live in discomfort and pain when you don't have to? Oftentimes, when medications allow you to feel some improvement and some sense that you can indeed get better, you gain a sense of encouragement and hopefulness that cannot be replaced. Once you make some headway in the level of pain and despair, there is so much more improvement that can be achieved with dietary and supplemental approaches. But if the medication provokes something else or makes symptoms worse, which can happen in a body that is already inflamed, communication with your prescriber is key.

Obviously, medications require prescriptions and therefore a physician, which can sometimes be an obstacle. Regardless, I think it important to share the full spectrum of what I offer patients because I have seen great benefits over the years. My two important integrative protocols are as follows. **Please keep in mind:** I am a medical doctor and a researcher, and I have carefully researched these protocols and talked with countless patients about their experience with them. They may work for you. But I am not *your* doctor. Your doctor knows your history and will be able to direct you on what is likely to be helpful for *you*, so be sure to consult with them and follow their instructions.

Neuroinflammatory Protocol

The central nervous system—the brain and the spinal cord—has its own unique immune system and therefore its own unique inflammatory response against anything that assaults it, such as a virus exposure. In fact, about 90 percent of the cells in the brain are glial cells, which are immune cells. Glial cells are present all the time, but when the immune response is intense, as it is for patients with PEIs, the need for glial cells spikes. When that happens, the marrow of the skull can help out by producing other cells that contribute to the immune response. And what that means, of course, is more inflammation.

When the central nervous system is inflamed, you may experience headaches, dizziness, and brain fog. Functions that support cognition and memory are slowed, and it's harder for the brain to store new memories. This protocol has been effective in treating those symptoms.

I. ORAL BETAHISTINE: This drug has action on both H_1 (weak agonist) and H_3 (antagonist) receptors in the central nervous system, which is unusual because most antihistamines target the H_1 and H_2 receptors. H_3 receptors are fairly unique to the central nervous system, and this medication can increase the release of acetycholine and serotonin, among other neurotransmitters. Because of its weak agonism of H_1 receptors, it can also increase histamine, but most patients are on classic H_1 and H_2 blockers, which are found over the counter. Betahistine is hard to find, insurance companies often won't pay for it, and it usually has to be compounded. Betahistine also has indirect effects of vasodilation and can improve vertigo and pressure or pain of the ears. It can be very beneficial in addressing the symptoms of patients with chronic illness.

2. ORAL LORAZEPAM: Lorazepam is an immediate-acting benzodiazepine and, like other benzodiazepines, can stabilize mast cells and reduce sympathetic surges commonly experienced by those suffering with chronic illnesses. Available by prescription only, it should only be used under the careful care of a physician and for a short time.

3. ORAL GINGKO BILOBA: Gingko biloba is a polyphenol (a chemical compound that occurs in plants) with antioxidant and anti-inflammatory properties, and through these actions it holds powerful neuroprotective and neurotherapeutic effects. Available over the counter.

4. ORAL PANAX GINSENG: This contains ginsenosides that have antioxidant and anti-inflammatory effects that protect against decreased oxygen supply and neural immune response. Available over the counter.

5. ORAL ASPIRIN: Aspirin is a nonsteroidal anti-inflammatory agent notable for its blockage of cyclooxygenase, and therefore it works as a powerful anti-inflammatory agent for both short- and long-term inflammation. It also stabilizes mast cells,

which may be the reason why it can counteract the inflammation caused by radiation. Finally, as a blood thinner, it improves the circulation of blood through organ systems, including the brain. While a prescription is not needed, you should let your physician know you are taking aspirin.

6. ORAL ATORVASTATIN: A statin (a prescription drug for lowering cholesterol) that can help reduce the damage to the lining of the blood vessels and hence limit the level of endothelial (pertaining to cells lining various organs and blood vessels) dysfunction, which can cause cells and other substances to stick against the lumen wall and form clumps, impair blood flow, and create further inflammation.

7. ORAL DOXYCYCLINE: A prescription antibiotic with not only antimicrobial activity but important anti-inflammatory properties, and that helps to modulate the level of certain enzymes that come from the mast cells and target components of the connective tissue.

8. ORAL QUERCETIN: A flavonoid that is widely found in foods but also available as a supplement that stabilizes the membranes of mast cells and reduces the release of histamine as well as other mediators.

9. ORAL LOW-DOSE NALTREXONE: A small dose of this prescription-only opioid antagonist reduces glial cell (the brain's immune cells) reactivity and therefore reduces neuroinflammation.

Mitochondrial Repair Protocol

Mitochondria are organelles inside every cell in our body, and as we learn in high school biology, they are the energy powerhouse of the cell. If the demand is too high on the mitochondria, as it very often is with these illnesses, then the body needs more of the raw ingredients required to help boost and support the important role of the mitochondria to provide energy to each cell. This protocol supplies those raw ingredients in the best form possible.

Mitochondria also create waste from their important work in the form of free radicals, and those free radicals can be toxic. Under normal circumstances, mitochondria have certain mechanisms to sweep up their own free radicals, like taking out the garbage. But when the demand is too high on them, they struggle to do this. They end up making too many free radicals and overwhelm their clean-up mechanisms. They cannot keep up, and their garbage starts piling up. This protocol can also help alleviate that burden.

1. UROLITHIN A, 500 MG TWICE A DAY: This natural compound improves the health of the mitochondria. Supplement available over the counter.
2. QUERCETIN, 500 MG TWICE A DAY: This flavonoid is widely found in foods but also available as a supplement that stabilizes the membranes of mast cells, reduces the release of histamine as well as other mediators, and minimizes burden on mitochondria. Supplement available over the counter.

3. **COENZYME Q10 (COQ10), 300 MG TWICE A DAY:** A coenzyme that is part of the electron transport chain (ETC) of the mitochondria, it is necessary for the generation of energy. Supplement available over the counter.

4. **VITAMIN E IN OIL, 2 OUNCES DAILY:** This lipid-soluble vitamin has powerful antioxidant properties to reduce the quantity of reactive oxygen species produced by the mitochondria. Supplement available over the counter.

5. **VITAMIN C, 1,000 MG PER DAY:** This vitamin helps to regulate the efficiency of oxidative phosphorylation performed by the ETC of the mitochondria and is also necessary for healing and recovery.

6. **GROMWELL (LITHOSPERMUM ERYTHRORHIZON):** One of my favorite supplements for mitochondrial protection, gromwell supports healthy mitochondrial function. Supplement available over the counter, though hard to find; you may have to go online to get it.

7. **RESVERATROL, 500 MG TWICE A DAY:** This polyphenol has multiple mitoprotective effects, including improving efficiency of mitochondria turnover and scavenging reactive oxygen species to reduce damage to the mitochondria, and it helps the formation of new mitochondria to improve response to inflammation. Supplement available over the counter.

8. **MINERALS SODIUM, POTASSIUM, CALCIUM, MAGNESIUM, IRON, ZINC, COPPER, MANGANESE, SELE-**

NIUM: These minerals are necessary cofactors for the complex enzymes of the mitochondria that are critical for the production of the energy molecules. All are available over the counter, and there are some liquid tinctures that contain the combination.

9. L-CARNITINE, 1,000 MG TWICE A DAY: This is important for moving fatty acids into the mitochondria to support lipid metabolism for energy production. Supplement available over the counter.

10. ALPHA-LIPOIC ACID, 200 MG TWICE A DAY: This works as an important cofactor to support optimal mitochondrial replication and production. Supplement available over the counter.

11. THEOPHYLLINE (RX), 200 MG TWICE A DAY: A prescription medication that can improve efficacy of oxidative phosphorylation; it is good for improved energy production.

12. OXALOACETATE, 1,000 MG TWICE A DAY: This plays an important role by supporting the substrate cycles for the mitochondria, thereby improving their function. Supplement available over the counter.

I should point out, too, that some medications from the old days are making a comeback and are being repurposed or repositioned for more modern symptoms and diseases, or at least a more modern understanding of the disease. Doctors have often used medications off-label, meaning for purposes other than what they were studied for or approved for, but because of known mechanisms of action it makes sense to try them with other diseases and different symptoms. Sometimes they work, and sometimes they don't. Since Covid and all the ensuing research, it has become increasingly clear that the immune system plays a critical role in all post-viral and post-exposure sequelae and syndromes, and the repurposing or repackaging of different immunotherapies has shown some promise. I for one have dived into trying many of these medications, most commonly some of the newer targeted immune therapies but also some of the old guard such as azathioprine, methotrexate, and cyclophosphamide, which are typically prescribed for cancers and rheumatoid arthritis.

When people hear the word "integrative," as in "integrative therapy" or "integrative medicine," they often think mainly of complementary treatments such as supplements, diet, acupuncture, yoga, and so on. But a truly integrative approach involves treating the whole self—your physical, mental, and emotional needs—through complementary as well as conventional, or allopathic, treatments. Medication, combined with a healthy diet and smart usage of supplements, can be a critical early step on your journey toward recovery.

Take-Home Guidelines

1. Avoid sugar and heavily processed foods, and increase consumption of whole foods, especially dark leafy greens and cruciferous vegetables. Consider juicing to optimize quantity of nutrients and vitamins.

2. Do not consume whole foods until ten A.M., and stop eating food after five P.M.
3. Do not consume more than one to two glasses of alcohol per week, go for a walk outside after a meal as it will reduce glucose blood spikes as well as further cravings, and drink hot lemon tea after each meal as this too will reduce the cravings for sugary foods.
4. Use supplements judiciously. Talk to your doctor about supplements you are taking or are planning on taking.
5. Talk to your doctor about what medications will help you. Try to get medications compounded if possible.

6

Movement and Movement Therapies

READ THIS CHAPTER TO FIND OUT . . .

- How to use activity and exercise to address your symptoms
- When to see a doctor or physical therapist
- What physical and manual therapies might be right for you

OUR BODIES ARE MEANT TO be in motion. In fact, regular physical activity is one of the most important things we can do for our health. It provides immediate benefits such as better cognition and reduced anxiety. It can help prevent various diseases such as type 2 diabetes, cardiovascular disease, and some kinds of cancer, and even reduce the impact of some infectious diseases, including Covid-19. It strengthens our bones and muscles, helps us manage our weight, and generally just makes us feel good.

Yet in our modern culture we spend most of our days sitting in a chair or couch, or lying in bed. We may exercise, but then we sit some more. When we're not sitting, we're looking for a place to sit. And that applies to those of us who are *not* chronically ill.

Of course, the increasing population of people who do have chronic and complex disease are unable to be active in any substantial manner. Mild exercise or even sometimes small movements can cause significant fatigue, prolonged recovery, and/or crashes, in which symptoms of pain, stimuli overload, weakness, and more are exacerbated. So we don't move as much as we need to, and that has a negative effect on our musculoskeletal and cardiovascular systems that further compounds the disease. We need to regularly recruit muscle and increase our heart rate and circulate our blood. When cells are forced to provide energy, they take up oxygen better. Blood flow is higher, and metabolic waste by-products are released and drained more easily. We build strength in the connection of the cells and thereby optimize the function of the organ. We get stronger, more agile, and increase our resilience. When we move our bodies, we connect with our bodies, and it is that connection that provides the intuition—or that sixth sense—of what our bodies need to be better in their position, how they take up space, and how we can move from point A to point B. It teaches us what our bodies can do. This leads to increased strength and stamina for both external and internal challenges. With higher reserves, we can better fight exposure assaults on our physical and physiological systems. We move, we live. We live, we move. Come what may, we are more equipped to handle it not only physically but mentally.

Chances are you understand all this, at least on a basic level, and perhaps you were once very fit and active, if not downright athletic, before chronic illness came along. Many of my patients have been in this boat. It is so hard for them to accept the idea that they can no longer engage in activity at a level they were used to before they got sick. Many of these patients, at the beginning of their illness when they first realized they could no longer regularly run as far, climb as high, or go as fast, sought evaluation by other physicians, who told them they were not as fit as they were because they are getting older, and that is what happens with aging.

"Aging" as a reason for why patients do not feel well is a common song from doctors, especially when the real cause of symptoms is elusive. It's convenient because the fact that we are getting older is true, and a patient can't argue with that. We are all getting older each day. But the idea that our symptoms are because of the aging process is not a valid one. I remember when I was in residency training, patients in their forties and fifties would come in with concerns that they could no longer exercise as they were used to—not as they used to in their twenties, mind you. They made it clear they were comparing to the way they were able to exercise a few months prior, despite no obvious change in their lifestyle. My attending would often tell them they were just getting older and would have to change their expectations of what their body should be expected to do, almost implying, "What do you expect?" But listening to their stories, it was clear to me they were picking up on the difference in how their bodies felt, moved, and performed. They knew it was different; they knew there was a change. And it was not because of their age. Or their gender.

Other invalid diagnoses include anxiety, depression, or, my personal favorite, perimenopause or menopause, an offensive explanation for why women present with concerns about their health. It is quite possible that a very early sign of chronic illness is a decrease in stamina and strength that is so subtle that only the person experiencing it can appreciate it, which is why there should be more focus on listening to the patient, because who else knows their body but the one who has lived in it for decades? All my medical school training and experience as a doctor does not give me the ability to sense what is happening in a patient's body more than they can. Listen to what your body is telling you.

Start Slow and Track the Effects

MOVEMENT IS A KEY TO recovery from chronic illness, especially for those symptoms related to connective tissue dysfunction (pages 52–56), but because of the chronic illness, movement can be very difficult. You may feel malaise and fatigue and even pain following decidedly small movements, and you are at risk of facing a prolonged period of recovery that can alter your life for days afterward. Movement under these circumstances will not only not be beneficial but could easily worsen the disease. What a lousy catch-22!

You may also feel held back from activity for emotional reasons. Many of my patients have felt hopelessness, frustration, or deep sadness about their inability to exercise or even be slightly active the way they used to. I will never forget one of my patients, a man named Nathan, who was a rock climber, or at least he had been. Mountain climbing and rock climbing were, he said, his greatest loves, and he had these incredibly thick fingers to prove it. His fingers had muscles. He said he could do pull-ups with his fingers when he was healthy. Wistfully, he told me about his adventures in Yosemite, Joshua Tree, and other places worldwide—adventures he referred to as his "past life" because they required physical strength and stamina that he could only dream of since he'd become ill. When he first came to me, Nathan was so sick that pretty much any activity at all was out of the question. He was not quite bedbound, but he was housebound for sure, and he was despondent. He said, "I need to move. It's who I am," but I had to caution him to hold back because I knew that trying to exercise would only make things worse for him. So we started with medicinal interventions, and eventually he started to have some better days mixed in with the bad ones. Then even better days, and more frequent good days. When he started having more good days than bad, it was time to try light exercise in his home; I still did not want him to leave home, and I told him not to use any weights and to do only three reps at a time. When we had our meetings online via telehealth he would report that he had followed my directions and was feeling okay, so I decided it was safe to add more reps, but still with no weights. When his reports continued to be positive, I told him to add one-pound weights, which he went online to buy and could only find in pink, which he complained about. "You can use pink hand weights," I said. "Who's going to see you?" We had a good laugh over that, and he used the weights, and slowly but surely we added more weights and more reps. Heavier hand weights, strap weights around his ankles. We took it very slowly, and sometimes he would tell me he was feeling some fatigue, and we would dial it back. I'd have him do two workouts this week instead of four. We stayed dialed in to how his body was feeling, and we tweaked his activity load as we went. And then one day nine or ten months later he messaged me that he had done the exercises with ten-pound weights, and he was crying. A man who regularly had scaled the faces of mountains. He had been so sick for so long, and his quality of life had degenerated so far, he felt he had lost his identity, but now he had done something he never thought he would be able to do again. It may sound like a small thing, working out with ten-pound weights, but it was not. It was a huge thing. And when I saw that message from Nathan, I knew for sure that he was on the road to recovery, because I could see that his hope had returned. I was so proud of him. I saw him for maybe two more years after that, and the last I heard from him he was taking some three-mile hikes, and he was feeling really good, and it was clear that he would keep getting better. I believe the difference was movement. He was on medication and made dietary changes and other changes, but it was the movement that helped him to trust his body again, believe in his recovery, and stay motivated.

If you're like Nathan and you are too weak to be active, or too depressed or emotionally exhausted, or physically exhausted, then you may have to wait on movement until you make some gains through pharmacological and other means. Again, you know your body best. If you can do small movements and minimal activity without further stressing your body, I recommend starting with short-duration walks each day. I ask you to not exert yourself too much, and while you may feel like you could do more, the best thing to do is do less and see how you feel the next day. When you feel like you can do more, do more. You don't have to climb Mount Everest or complete an Ironman competition to get benefits from movement and exercise. In addition to short walks, you can do yoga, Pilates, or Gyrotonic (more on this later). You can do weight lifting or bicycle riding or take an aerobics class. The point is if you feel like you can move, then move. But take it slowly and wait to see how you respond to that activity, and track how you feel so you can have more insight into how to do it differently, or if at all. It can be key to regularly check in with your body, because if you find you can do more—even a little—on one day versus another, that can be important information that can help with your treatment.

Tracking how you feel is important, especially early on. I recommend using a journal to record how long you spent on one activity; how you felt before, during, and after the activity; and how you felt the next day. It does not have to be elaborate, you don't have to write long journal entries, and you certainly don't have to be Hemingway. You might even make a spreadsheet with columns for "Duration," "How I felt before," "How I felt during," "How I felt after," and "How I felt the next day" and jot down notes. After a while you may be able to identify a trend or triggers. Maybe short walks outside are consistently making you feel better and think a bit more clearly, but yoga, especially moves that involve bending upside down, leads to headaches. In that case, you might want to focus on longer or more frequent walks and cut back on yoga for a while (or limit it to upright poses). Understanding how your body feels and responds to any minimal activity or task can give insight into how best to structure and plan a day. It is also a way of getting in tune with your body and connecting with it again so that you can help nurture and support your body and brain during recovery.

I also recommend monitoring certain parameters to get a sense of how your body physiologically responds to any activity you are able to engage in—whether it be walking, stretching, or even cooking, cleaning, dressing, and showering. Parameters to record in the journal include:

- Heart rate
- Blood pressure
- Respiratory rate
- Pulse oxygen saturation levels
- Glucose levels

It's important to empower ourselves with this information, and you can get it for a fairly low cost. You can get a smart watch like a Fitbit for relatively cheap, many of which will track heart rate, respiratory rate, and oxygen levels. Your doctor can prescribe a continuous glucose monitor, and you can use finger-stick glucose checkers found in the drugstore if need be. You can get a blood pressure monitor for the home for less than a hundred dollars. Taken together, these devices put a lot of data at your fingertips that tells you about your body and what your body is doing and how it is responding to different activities and interventions.

As with your journal entries about activity, you are looking for trends. For example, anyone can have an elevated heart rate at any given point—there are various reasons for it—but if your heart rate remains elevated, and you don't feel well, you should seek care from your primary doctor.

Similarly, if you find that a change in heart rate is correlated with a certain symptom, such as headaches, fatigue, or dizziness, that is information that you will want to tell your doctor. It is the same with all the other parameters. Something trending one way or another gives you a marker that something is out of balance, something acute might be happening, and it's time to go to the doctor so you have a chance to get it under control. Monitoring glucose levels can give you a gross estimate of your body's metabolic response to all activities as well as physiological states such as hunger, satiety, stress, drowsiness, and sleep. The more data, the better for understanding how your body responds not only to external stimuli but to internal as well. Again, ultimately these data points serve as important insights into how your body is objectively responding to different activities, food, sleep quality, medications, exposures, stress, and more.

I should note that many with chronic illness eventually may stop having the classic objective or obvious physiological change to external or even internal stimuli as the body just sort of accommodates, but it doesn't mean that the disease does not exist. A good example is when those with low intracranial pressure suffer from what is called orthostatic headaches, whereby they experience severe headaches when they stand up. Over time, those headaches are no longer just when they stand, and often the severity of the waxing and waning of the headaches lessens. But they still have low intracranial pressure.

If, after being active, you find that you are not able to do minimal activity or exertion, you will want to find a physical therapist who is literate and intimately familiar with connective tissue and its functions, and who offers home visits or video visits. Post-exertional malaise is a cornerstone of chronic fatigue syndrome but can occur with fibromyalgia and other chronic diagnoses, so it is important to slowly evaluate your response to movement and adjust accordingly. A good physical therapist can help provide some simple, safe, and gentle stretches or movement that can be done while lying in bed or sitting in a chair. You will read more about physical therapists and movement therapy on pages 180–187.

Suggested Exercises

AS YOU BUILD UP YOUR strength from these first slow steps, it won't be long before you're able to do a bit more. And then more after that. This not only feels great, but it continues your healing process. Below are a few exercises I recommend to help your body help itself heal.

When you work out, try to remember not to always start exercises on the same side. If you are right-handed, for example, it is always tempting and usually reflexive to start exercises with your right arm or right leg and then do the left, but over time this can be detrimental, because it can cause an imbalance in the central nervous system. When we are chronically inflamed, we need to retrain our bodies on many different levels. Even beyond exercise, be cognizant of your handedness habits, and reach for that doorknob with your nondominant hand, eat with your nondominant hand. When you ascend stairs, step with your nondominant leg first. This kind of "cross activity" recruits the opposite side of the brain, helps to retrain the neural system, and helps balance out your overall fitness, health of muscles and nerves, and your feelings of recovery. Many neurological diseases such as Parkinson's disease present unilaterally, or on one side of the body, and it may be important to be mindful of challenging your nondominant side.

Morning Twist

When you wake up in the morning, get up slowly from the bed. Abruptly jumping out of bed can easily cause injury and damage to tissue. Also, studies have shown that heart attacks and strokes often happen in the early morning hours due to the sudden exertion.

Roll to your side in bed, sit up, place your feet on the floor, take five deep breaths, and allow your body to calibrate. Then stand slowly and stretch your arms out and lift them overhead. With your arms extended overhead, turn your torso slightly to the right, and then back to center. Then turn your torso slightly to the left, and then back to center. Repeat.

Stand on One Foot

Stand on one foot for ten seconds. You do not have to lift your foot up high—stay within your means so the risk of falling is very low. You can lift one foot as high as the opposite ankle, or even rest it on the ankle. You can be by a chair or the wall in case you need to hold on. After doing one foot for ten seconds, repeat on the other side.

Shrug and Roll

While standing on stable ground, lift your shoulders to your ears and then lower them back down with a backward roll of the shoulder to a space that feels good to your body and posture. Do this ten times.

Rise Up

Stand from a sitting position without the use of your arms or hands.

Elbows Back

While standing on stable ground, bring your hands to meet each other in front of your chest with your elbows out to your sides. Then move your elbows backward as far as they can go while pushing your sternum (chest) outward. This helps realign the sternum with the rib cage and engages the back muscles.

Gyrotonic Method

I'm a huge proponent of the Gyrotonic system. If you haven't heard of it, it is a way of exercising the joints through circular movements using a weight and pulley system. Whenever someone has a connective tissue problem, joints are affected, so it's imperative that patients focus on movements that target joints. The Gyrotonic movements are remarkably effective at keeping joints flexible, strong, and stable, and they strengthen muscles that support joints. When people hear the word "joints," they commonly think of shoulders, elbows, or knees, but remember that the spine is a series of joints, and it is central to the healing journey of many patients with post-exposure illnesses. Walking and other low-impact exercises are definitely helpful, but the Gyrotonic system is specifically designed to recruit several different joints at the same time, like a little choreography for your joints.

The problem with the Gyrotonic system, of course, is that you do need a machine to engage in it—as well as a teacher—and it can be a challenge to find these. Some physical therapists have the machines, and in some cities you can find dedicated Gyrotonic studios. It's a new but quickly growing exercise, so even if you don't have access to Gyrotonic now, you may soon. If you are lucky enough to have access to Gyrotonic, I can't recommend it highly enough.

If Gyrotonic is not an option for you right now, you do have some alternatives you can do at home for free. While not as thorough as Gyrotonic, they can offer real benefit.

I recommend regular gentle yoga, especially the child's pose. Sit with your butt on your heels, then bend forward at the waist, keeping your butt on your heels. Rest your forehead on the floor. You can put your arms palm down on the floor in front of you or reach back so they're next to your legs, palms up. Hold for several seconds or longer. This is a great pose for stretching your hip flexors and spine.

An even better option is to see a physical therapist who specializes in people with joint hypermobility. You can even get great benefit from PTs on social media, such as on Instagram or YouTube. One of my favorites is Melissa Koehl.

Movement for Post-Surgical Patients

CRANIOCERVICAL FUSION SURGERY HELPS TO resolve the symptoms that come from instability of the craniocervical joint, which connects the base of the skull to the first two joints of the spine. Instability in this joint can cause compression of the lower part of the brainstem and can compress cranial nerves and vessels. This can cause headaches, dizziness, ringing of the ears, and feeling like you are going to pass out. Some patients even do pass out. Patients with PEI can develop craniocervical instability because of the inflammation and the release of enzymes and other mediators that is so characteristic of PEIs. Some of these mediators attack the connective tissue and affect the ligaments that are holding that crucial joint together.

If you have had surgery to correct craniocervical instability, tethered cord, or any spinal problem, whether it is instability of other parts of the cervical spine, disc herniation, Chiari malformation, spondylolisthesis, or spinal stenosis, you may naturally have concerns about what movement to do and when you can start. Initially after surgery, be extra careful and minimize movement, but within three to seven days, depending on any coexisting health challenges you may have had pre-surgery or the extent to which you have lost conditioning, it is important to start to challenge the body. You might expect that you'd want to strengthen the spine and the accessory spinal muscles, but in chronic illness patients that could potentially slow down recovery and even cause a flare of symptoms because it can move a spinal cord that has been under tension and compromised for multiple years prior to the intervention to correct it.

I am not an exercise physiologist, but I have spent years helping, guiding, and learning from post-operative patients, and I have gained tremendous insight into how best to support their immediate post-operative recovery in terms of physical activity and movement. And while I know many surgeons and physical therapists will have patients up and doing back-strengthening exercises, I often recommend starting with the small peripheral muscles, such as your hands and feet. Peripheral exercises indirectly recruit core and paraspinal muscles and are safer for a post-operative spine. Here are a few exercises to start with. Start with lighter weights and gradually increase the resistance as you get stronger. It's also important to maintain proper form and technique to avoid injury.

Hammer Curls

Hold a pair of dumbbells with a neutral grip (palms facing each other) and let your arms hang straight down at your sides. Keeping your upper arms stationary, curl the weights up at the same time toward your shoulders while keeping your wrists in a neutral position.

Reverse Curls

Hold a barbell with an overhand grip (palms facing down) and let your arms hang straight down at your sides. Keeping your upper arms stationary, curl the barbell up toward your shoulders while keeping your wrists in that overhand position.

Supination and Pronation

Hold a dumbbell with an underhand grip (palms facing up) and let your arm hang straight down at your side. Keeping your upper arm stationary, rotate your wrist and forearm outward (supination), and then rotate them back inward (pronation).

Calf Raises

Stand with your feet hip-width apart and place your hands on a wall or a sturdy object for support. Slowly rise up onto the balls of your feet, lifting your heels as high as possible. Hold for a moment at the top, then lower your heels back down to the starting position. Repeat for several repetitions.

Jump Rope

Jumping rope is a great cardiovascular exercise that also engages your calf muscles. Start with a regular jump rope and jump continuously, aiming to keep a steady rhythm. As you jump, focus on pushing off the balls of your feet and engaging your calf muscles to propel yourself upward.

Calf Stretches

Stretching your calves is important for maintaining flexibility and preventing tightness. One effective calf stretch is the standing calf stretch. Stand facing a wall with one foot in front of the other, and place your hands on the wall for support. Keeping your back leg straight, gently lean forward, feeling the stretch in your calf. Hold for about thirty seconds, then switch legs.

Calf Raises on a Stair

Stand on the edge of a step or a sturdy platform with your heels hanging off the edge. Hold on to a railing or a wall for support. Lower your heels down below the step, then push up onto your tiptoes, lifting your heels as high as you can. Lower back down and repeat for several repetitions. I generally say to repeat as tolerated to keep patients from overdoing it, but the range is usually between four and ten repetitions.

Gentle Post-Surgical Stretching Routine

GENTLE STRETCHING CAN ALSO HELP keep things limber and slow down scar formation, which is an enemy of an EDS body because the unreliable integrity of the connective tissue makes healing difficult; many patients with EDS form not only abnormal scars but excessive scar tissue and have a propensity to develop thick scar tissue from surgery. The following routine is a good place to start. Do it several times a day, especially in between exercises, and soon you will be able to ramp up to more demanding movement. These stretching exercises can help promote flexibility and aid in the recovery process.

Gentle Range of Motion Exercises

The point with these exercises is to move the affected body part through its full range of motion. For example, if you had knee surgery, you might start with gentle knee bends and extensions to improve flexibility. Perform these exercises slowly and within your comfort level.

Passive Stretching

Passive stretching involves using an external force, such as a strap or a towel, to gently stretch the muscles. This can be helpful for increasing flexibility and preventing muscle stiffness. Make sure to perform these stretches in a controlled and pain-free manner.

Deep Breathing with Stretching

Deep breathing exercises can help relax the body and promote blood flow. As you inhale, gently stretch the affected area or surrounding muscles. For example, if you had shoulder surgery, take a deep breath and gently raise your arm, focusing on maintaining a relaxed and controlled movement.

The Relationship Between Anatomy and Health

WHEN WE START MEDICAL SCHOOL, we spend six months in gross anatomy and dissect cadavers assigned to us. I was always touched by the idea that people, during their lives, thought highly enough about science and medical education to agree to let first-year medical students congregate over their corpse and dissect it piece by piece, all for the sake of learning what the human body is made of.

I remember my cadaver well. I shared her with the three other medical students in my group. It was my first time seeing a dead body, and even though I have seen many more since that time, I will never forget her. Her name was Cathy, and she had died of a heart attack at the age of seventy-six. She had a pacemaker that our scalpels struck as we dissected into her sternum. Her toenails and fingernails were painted pink; those manicured nails were particularly meaningful to me because they represented her life prior to her death. She took time to care for herself, had preferences for her look, and was feminine. In some respects, Cathy represented what I had come to see in hospitals throughout my training and practice, wherein family members place pictures of the patient during better days on the wall of their hospital room in an attempt to get the doctors and care team to see who this patient was before they became the sick person in the hospital bed— a real person with loved ones, interests, and a full life. It was impactful and meaningful to me.

While dissecting Cathy, we took great effort to learn every nerve, muscle, vessel, organ, tendon, ligament, gland, duct, and bone in preparation for the weekly exams we were subject to. These exams were stressful, and we were grateful to have Cathy to study on. The anatomists who were our instructors would place a blank white label with an arrow pointing at a particular piece of anatomy on each cadaver, and we students had to go from table to table and name what the label was pointing at. For the most part, anatomical pieces are in similar locations in everyone, but their ratio to other anatomical pieces—which is sometimes the basis for naming them—can be slightly or even more than slightly different from one body to the next. And sometimes they were found somewhere else in the body completely, something we call ectopic or an anomaly. With no medical history on the bodies that were assigned to us for our study, we were left to discover when there was a piece of the body missing or in a different location, ultimately making the entire region unfamiliar, since much of the learning of anatomy is based on landmarks. If you first locate anatomy structure A, then you look in this direction and you will find anatomy structure B, and so on.

During those six months, we could not appreciate just how critical this anatomy is to the thousands of biochemical and physiological reactions that take place within this body. We had separate courses on biochemistry where we focused on how the body handles macronutrients and micronutrients and creates energy and other important compounds. We also had courses on normal physiology, where we learned how the lungs breathe, the heart beats, the muscles move, the liver detoxifies, the kidneys filter, and so on. We then delved into different organ systems and learned disease and pathophysiology, which is basically the study of what goes wrong and why, and what symptoms a patient may have and what treatments we can try. There was the heavy neuroscience course where we learned a completely different language and had a separate lab to learn the anatomical regions of the brain.

In other words, in all this learning we did to become well-trained doctors, we never discussed the idea that anatomy could play a critical role in health and disease. The curriculum focused on organ systems, and we tackled one organ at a time and delved into all the different diseases and the pathophysiology associated with that organ itself. There was some discussion of the intersection between organs, depending on the disease, but the anatomical relationships between organs or within the rest of the human framework was not thought to be relevant to the study of disease.

But it is relevant and highly pertinent. The more I practice, the more I realize that our structural and mechanical bodies may very well be directing our physiological health. It is obvious to see that misalignment of a joint—say a dislocation or subluxation of the shoulder or the knee—can cause pain and dysfunction. Who can move their arm if their shoulder is dislocated? But so much is intertwined with anatomy, and everything is connected. Rib subluxation (partial dislocation) can cause difficulty for the lungs to expand and dyskinesia (jerky, clunky movements) in the diaphragm. Shoulder dislocation can affect the brachial plexus, which is a configuration of nerves that feed the muscles of our shoulder, upper back, and entire arm. These are simple examples.

If you take the connective tissue as a collective unit and

realize it functions as its own organ and recognize it quite literally holds things together—and holds them where they should be for proper functioning—it's easy to understand the sheer magnitude of the importance of alignment. Move the uterus or bladder in one direction, and the intestines are redistributed. If the spine curves, as it does in scoliosis, very commonly seen with connective tissue disorders, the nerve roots traverse a less conventional path and resort to a perhaps tortuous or winding connection to their outpost, changing the messaging ever so slightly. An even mildly altered nerve path can result in numbness or pain in an extremity, weakness or paralysis, persistent headaches, or worse.

The point is that the body relies on its structure—specifically, its structure where all pieces are in their appropriate spots. And more specifically, spots that optimize the relationships between the organs and tissues. Because we are one whole organism, and everything is connected either directly or indirectly—each cell, each tissue, each connecting fiber relies on the interconnectedness of the whole. It is a network of active, bustling communication pathways, and when communication along one of those pathways is interrupted, messages don't get received. If a message is left hanging long enough, the sender—whether it's an organ or a system—will stop thinking it is necessary and stop trying to send it. If that pathway is not reactivated at some point in the near future, it begins to degenerate. When that happens, we may experience all sorts of symptoms such as pain, fatigue, tremulousness (shaking or quivering), malaise, numbness, tingling, difficulty with movement, and other symptoms based on which organ system is involved. When healthy, the connective tissue prevents things like that from happening. The importance of connective tissue cannot be overstated.

Physical and Manual Therapies

SO WHEN CONNECTIVE TISSUE BREAKS down or is compromised, as is often the case in patients with chronic post-exposure illness, and perhaps things are starting to get misaligned, what can be done? You actually have a very accessible and effective treatment available to you. What seems so ominous and tragic can actually be mostly prevented with regular and consistent physical and manual therapies, especially when started early. I tell my patients with any kind of connective tissue compromise that physical therapy is and always will be a cornerstone of their preventive and therapeutic care.

If you have connective tissue dysfunction, seek out a therapist who is literate in hypermobility and its common co-occurring conditions such as craniocervical instability and MCAS, and establish a regular physical therapy schedule and corresponding home exercises as directed by the therapist. The exercises are meant to maintain flexibility of joints but also to improve strength of the muscles supporting the joints, challenge and strengthen vestibular and balance function, and create safe movement for your body, which promotes better blood flow and the movement of lymph—a fluid that carries white blood cells as a critical part of the immune system—through the body. It can also help to restore an internal milieu so messages are not being dropped, thus helping to keep your body working in a balanced way.

Regarding post-operative physical therapy, specifically for CCI, tethered cord (TC), or other spinal surgery for common spinal pathologies of the EDS patient population, it's important to remember to hold off on recruiting the muscles of the back and those supporting the spine too quickly. Start by exercising peripheral muscles first, as described on page 171, and work slowly toward your center as you build strength, stamina, and health. As for other surgeries, physical therapy guidelines may be tailored based on the surgery and the original indication for the surgery.

Once you have engaged in physical therapy for a period of time, approximately six to twelve months, manual therapies can be incorporated for deeper realignment and musculoskeletal stability work. Our vertebrae and their intersecting cartilaginous discs are designed to accommodate the total burden of all that we do—standing, walking, bending, twisting, sitting, and so on—and distribute it along the total length of the spine. The spine is held tight and strong by the muscles and connective tissue that surround it. Over time, with chronic inflammation, trauma, or congenital connective tissue dysfunction, the spine can lose strength and integrity and fall out of alignment. If this process starts when someone is young and still growing, it can cause a curvature of the spine, called scoliosis, which can further impose burden on the whole spine, including the spinal cord and its nerves.

The joints of the spine do not dislocate or subluxate in the classic sense as with other joints, but they do slip off of each other, called listhesis. The discs can bulge or, worse, herniate, meaning they protrude from within the spinal column. While one is an embryo developing in utero, the notochord, which is the early spine, serves as a conductor of sorts in directing where and how other cells migrate and differentiate, and what organ they become. The notochord is ultimately replaced by the spine, but you can see how this piece of embryology points to how this structure can dictate the entire topography of the body. Protecting this part of our skeleton is a key element of allowing our bodies to move and take up space in positions where organ systems can sit comfortably with one another. Part of that care includes manual therapies, because manual therapy can help move things into place.

Manual therapy is a type of physical therapy in which a clinician applies hands-on techniques to manipulate soft tissue, joints, and nerves to decrease pain and tissue tension and improve quality of movement. This can optimize blood flow, reduce inflammation, and reduce stress and strain on joints and soft tissue. You can likely have any of the following manual therapies performed by your physical therapist, if you have one, but you may also find another specialist, such as an occupational therapist, massage therapist, or athletic trainer. When searching for a manual therapy clinician, look for one who is licensed by your state.

Cranial Sacral Therapy

One important manual therapy is cranial sacral therapy, in which a therapist applies gentle pressure on the head, neck, and back to relieve the stress and pain caused by compression in the bones of the head, sacrum (a triangular bone in the lower back), and spinal column. Cranial sacral therapy can help move lymph through the dura, the membrane that envelops the brain and spinal cord, and enhance movement of cerebrospinal fluid as well. It helps support supple and stable mobility of the joints of the spine.

If you have symptoms of back pain, headaches, lightheadedness, or fatigue, I recommend getting cranial sacral therapy once a week as an adjunct therapy. Cranial sacral therapy can help relieve muscle spasms and indirect pressure on nerves as well as reduce inflammation in connective tissues. It can further support realignment temporarily.

Myofascial Release Therapy

Myofascial release is a therapy in which the therapist gently massages the fascia, the tissues that encase our muscle bundles throughout our body. Myofascial release is mainly used on non-axial muscles—those of our limbs. It helps to release tension held in the fascia, which is important because when our spine is failing, as can happen with connective tissue dysfunction, our limbs take up the slack to keep us from crumbling into a heap. The muscles can constrict and spasm, often in response to aberrant signaling from the nerves that emanate from the spinal cord to speak to the muscles of our limbs. Releasing the fascia helps to release muscle tension and allow for more fluid movement, reduced pain, and improved structural integrity of the muscle tissue. Acupressure, the use of palpation at certain convergent points of our anatomy, can be very effective for this as well.

I recommend myofascial release therapy once a week for anyone who has indications of connective tissue dysfunction. Myofascial release is a great form of therapy to minimize the effects of the diffuse muscular spasm causing pain and decreased range of motion and mobility for patients with connective tissue compromise due to either genetic or acquired disorders.

Lymphatic Massage

I would be remiss if I did not discuss the incredible benefits many of my patients receive from regular lymphatic massage. These specialized massages are designed to accomplish effective and efficient drainage of the lymph, which has a very positive impact on the immune system. The lymphatic system is a network of vessels and organs situated beneath the skin that acts something like a garbage disposal system, helping your body filter out waste and bacteria. Stagnation of lymph can occur with chronic, perpetual inflammatory responses to infectious agents, mold, toxic substances, chronic diseases such as diabetes, hypertension, obesity, and even from chronic insomnia, chronic poor nutrition, lack of exercise and movement, and more, and it compromises the body's response to these assaults. Stagnation also happens with anatomical misalignment, as we so often see with connective tissue compromise. Lymphatic massage uses gentle pressure to coax lymph from inflamed tissues to functioning lymph nodes, therefore helping to drain the body of toxins. Lymphatic massage also helps the brain to release waste and debris, so clearance overall is improved, helping to reduce inflammation.

For an optimal lymphatic massage, seek out a well-trained therapist who understands the planes of the lymphatic system and its directional flow toward the lymph nodes, based on the region of the body. But you can also do some basic lymphatic massage on your own. If you're getting massage from a therapist, I recommend getting treatment once a week. If you're doing it yourself, you can do it two or three times a week. Whenever you have lymphatic massage, be sure to drink plenty of water afterward. You may also need to rest: Pay attention to how your body feels, and rest accordingly. Lymphatic massage is not recommended for people who have a heart condition, kidney problems, or cellulitis.

Here is a routine to help you get started with lymphatic massage:

1. **FIND A COMFORTABLE POSITION.** Sit or lie down in a comfortable position, ensuring that your body is relaxed and supported.
2. **START AT THE NECK.** Gently place your fingertips on the sides of your neck, just below your ears. Use gentle, rhythmic motions to massage downward toward the collarbone. Repeat this motion several times, gradually moving along the sides of your neck.
3. **MOVE TO THE ARMPITS.** Place your hands on your armpits and use gentle circular motions to massage the area. This is where many lymph nodes are located, so massaging this area can help facilitate lymphatic drainage. Repeat this motion for a few minutes.
4. **MASSAGE THE CHEST.** With your fingertips, make small circles on your chest, starting from the center and moving outward toward the sides. Be gentle and avoid applying excessive pressure.
5. **MASSAGE TOWARD THE HEART.** It is important to always massage in the direction of the heart to encourage lymphatic flow. This means moving your hands or fingers from your extremities toward your torso.

Exposure to cold can be adjuvant as it constricts the lymphatic vessels and aids movement of the lymph through the vessels toward the nodes. This can be as simple as a cold shower before and after or ice packs briefly applied to the focal area of your massage.

Connections

IT ALWAYS AMAZES ME HOW there can be a domino effect when we start to work on one highway of the body, and the intersecting highways seem to open up with less traffic and congestion and therefore less road rage, again pointing to the intricate interconnectedness within us. A symptom may present and worsen because of something happening upstream or downstream, perhaps even several steps removed from the root cause. We don't know until we look at one thing at a time to find that root cause, but there is no doubt that in the meantime there is a lot we can do to start cleaning up those roadways and the off-ramps and get things moving.

Manual and movement therapies take the body as a whole and move it about, literally and figuratively. The body was designed to move, but various obstacles on the path of life can interfere with its ability to do so, at least in a holistic and beneficial manner. A well-trained therapist can help in so many great ways. Not only do these therapies aid in wellness and health and recovery, but it feels good and gives you a boost in confidence that your body can indeed work for you.

I know that many of you reading may not be able to move much right now, and this talk of moving and exercising, and even getting up and going to a physical therapist, may sound like a cruel tease. But I believe movement is so important that I must urge you to do what you can. Start somewhere. Even the most severely affected patients can try to move their bodies, and you will feel better when you do. You may not be able to work out for an hour, but if you start somewhere, even moving legs and arms on the bed, the couch, or while in a chair, you can build from that place, wherever it is, and you will remember how good it feels to move. So I hope you will not feel like I'm being insensitive, because I absolutely know how you feel, and I hope you will not feel that this chapter does not apply to you, because it absolutely does. I do not give up on any of my patients. I believe in you.

Take-Home Guidelines

1. Moving is healing! But if you're feeling bad due to chronic illness, it can be hard to move much. Start slowly, and don't overdo it. Build up from there.
2. Track how you feel before, during, and after activity. Look for trends that might need to be addressed. (Or trends that show progress!)
3. Track your health parameters, again looking for trends. See your doctor if an indicator trends in the

wrong direction and especially if you feel symptoms related to changes in heart rate, blood pressure, or oxygen saturation.

4. Our anatomy is precise and depends on connective tissue to keep it that way. Therefore, physical therapy and rehabilitation medicine physicians to correct imbalance or connective tissue dysfunction can be key to your recovery.

5. Take things a step further with select manual therapies.

7

Oxygen and Breathing

READ THIS CHAPTER TO FIND OUT . . .

- How deliberate breathing can help with your chronic symptoms
- How to do simple breathing exercises
- The benefits of oxygen therapy
- The even greater benefits of going outside

WE NEED OXYGEN. OUR TISSUES need oxygen. Our cells need oxygen. Cellular machinery cannot function without oxygen.

Okay, so you don't need a neurologist to tell you that. But because breathing is an autonomic function, meaning our bodies do it without our having to think about it, well, we don't think about it. We know that we have some limited control over our breathing patterns—we hold our breath when we swim, we do deep breathing to settle ourselves when nervous or stressed or to get rid of hiccups (good luck with that)—but for the most part we take our breath for granted.

We take breathing so much for granted, in fact, that we often shortchange it. We rush, we worry, and we don't sleep well, and this all contributes to rapid, shallow breathing. Even under not-so-stressed circumstances, we don't tend to breathe deeply enough and therefore we don't get enough oxygen. Well, we get *enough*, strictly speaking. If you're reading this, you're alive. You may even check your oxygen saturation level and find that your readings are fine. But those readings measure a peripheral oxygen saturation level, and it is the *functionality* of oxygen that requires deeper appreciation. The penetration of the oxygen into the organ tissues, called perfusion, and the uptake and incorporation into the enzymatic processes of the oxygen molecules, called utilization, are often in deficit. Our breathing patterns and the force with which we breathe can play a role in the exchange of oxygen and carbon dioxide as well as blood flow movement and perfusion. It is one thing to have our blood deliver the oxygen to various tissues, but if it cannot perfuse from the vessel into the tissue, it does not offer as much benefit. This can alter other autonomic functions of the body, including the pulse, which further dictates flow and pressure of not only blood but cerebrospinal fluid. It can also affect our brain's restoration during sleep.

Our typically shallow and rapid breathing patterns can still saturate the hemoglobin with oxygen, making those measured saturation levels look okay, but they are not enough to move blood efficiently through the body.

Oxygen and Chronic Illness

DEFICITS ASSOCIATED WITH SHALLOW AND rapid breathing are common to many people. But they are magnified in the context of chronic illness, especially when characterized by dysfunction of the autonomic systems that affect our heart rate and breathing patterns, or by chronic inflammation due to exposures. The inflammatory mediators and the cells they recruit to help do battle against infection like to gather along the sides of the vessel walls, which results in the vessel wall becoming ragged, with divots and sticky spots where more cells collect and disrupt flow. It now requires more force for the oxygen, and the nutrients that accompany it in the blood, to cross the lining of the vessels and enter the cells of the tissue. It is like the defensive linemen trying to penetrate the offensive linemen protecting the quarterback—the quarterback being the tissue, of course.

Limited perfusion, and thus a lack of oxygen, is bad for any organ, but especially the brain. When the brain experiences a lack of oxygen, known as hypoxia, it shuts down some function to save energy; the result of that is not always extreme or obvious to an outsider, including a doctor, and may not show up in standard cognitive testing or other workups. It may result in a subtle change that the patient might experience as brain fog, or a sluggishness in their thinking, or even headaches. (Even when testing does not reveal any deficit, the patient knows. The patient always knows.) Hypoxic conditions cause accumulation of toxic by-products, headaches, seizures, cognitive decline, and more.

Luckily, there are some pretty straightforward ways to address hypoxia, starting with simply being more deliberate about our breathing. Stop, look, and breathe. I recommend, several times a day, to sit and focus on your breath:

- How deep are you inhaling?
- How long does it take to exhale?
- Does your chest rise?
- Does your abdomen rise?
- Do you breathe in or out through your nose or mouth?

Similarly, take some time daily to do some deep breathing. When we inhale deeply, we not only give pressure to blood flow circulating through our system, but we also increase the force or flow of cerebrospinal fluid. Force and velocity are also important for perfusion as well as lymphatic movement, which means our deep inhales and slow exhales help clear out inflammatory mediators and alleviate neuroinflammation overall.

Breathing patterns are also a way of connecting with and modulating the autonomic nervous system, which controls things like our heart rate, blood pressure, respiration, and digestion. Deep, deliberate breathing stimulates parasympathetic tone (the "rest and digest" function of our nervous system) to counteract the disproportionate sympathetic ("fight or flight") function that is usually predominant when we have lots of inflammation. It can also help regulate heart rate, which is commonly volatile in patients with PEIs. With deep and slow inspiration, the heart rate will go up, and with slow exhalation the heart rate will go down. These practices can help to overcome an acute autonomic flare of sympathetic surge, and when the fear and stress of your illness get the best of you, breath work can even help bring you back to center to think rationally about what can be done next.

Other Breathing Exercises

A MEASURED, FOCUSED APPROACH TO our inhalation can produce real physiological effects and go a long way toward supporting healing for anyone, but especially people with a chronic post-exposure illness. In fact, I think deep breath work is critical. Here are a couple exercises to help you achieve that goal.

Connect Your Breath to Movement

In the last chapter, you read about the importance of movement to health and recovery, and of course that is connected to oxygen and breathing. Many patients who struggle with chronic disease don't only have challenges with intentional movement, but they also tend to breathe more shallowly. With shallow breathing we don't draw in enough oxygen, and we also don't release enough carbon dioxide, the waste gas from respiration, so much so that carbon dioxide can accumulate within our blood, which can further complicate our natural breathing patterns as well as interfere with our sleep patterns.

This may sound abstract, but bear with me. Try to connect your breath to your movement. If you have done yoga, Pilates, or the Gyrotonic system, you have probably heard a trainer or instructor give directions to do just that. They may tell you to breathe out as you're moving this way, breathe in as you center again, breathe out as you move the other way, and so on. Or if you lift weights, you exhale as you lift and inhale as you lower. What I am suggesting is that you do this in your regular life. Control your breath.

You can do this in any area of your life, and the more often you do it the better. If you're unloading the dishwasher, inhale as you bend down to the rack (even if you have to hold on to the counter as you move your body), and give a long exhale as you stand up with the tray of silverware in hand. When you stand up from the desk or the couch, exhale deliberately and slowly as you do. If you're walking the dog, you can time your breathing with your steps: *In-two-three, out-two-three, in-two-three, out-two-three*. Even when speaking, try to control your breath. Be deliberate in your actions throughout the day, and by focusing on your breathing you will be able to ensure, as best as possible, abrupt changes of autonomic activity.

As I said, it's a bit abstract, and it's okay if you don't totally get it. It's a lot to think about, but the goal is to do just that: Think about your breathing. Get used to your breathing so you're in tune with it, and control it with deep breaths when you can, particularly when you can connect it with movements.

4–7–8 Breathing Exercise

This is probably my favorite breathing exercise, and it's a great one to do when you are feeling anxious, stressed, or overwhelmed. It is referred to as 4–7–8 breathing, and I first learned it in 2008 from Dr. Andrew Weil.[1] I recommend it to all my patients, and I use it frequently myself.

Sit quietly in a quiet room with your hands on your knees. Take note of how you are breathing and feeling at that moment. Then follow these steps:

1. Breathe in slowly for **four** counts through your nose with your mouth closed.

---

1 Andrew Weil, "Breathing Exercises: 4–7–8 Breath," Weil, https://www.drweil.com/videos-features/videos/breathing-exercises-4–7–8-breath/.

2. At the end of the inhale, with the tip of your tongue on the roof of your mouth behind your front teeth, hold your breath for **seven** counts.
3. Keeping your tongue in the same place, open your mouth and breathe out slowly through your mouth for **eight** counts.
4. Repeat up to ten times.

Many have noted how easy it is to rebalance and calm oneself with this breathing exercise. Many have also noted a decrease in heart rate at the end of the exercise. I have regularly measured blood pressure in the clinic during this exercise, and there is most certainly a beneficial effect on both heart rate and blood pressure as well as overall presence and energy.

Oxygen Therapy

I'M A HUGE FAN OF oxygen therapy as a way to help patients make gains that last. After pharmacological interventions and perhaps movement, oxygen therapy is probably the most critical path to improvement, and what's great is that even bedbound patients can do some forms of it. Oxygen is a well-regarded acute treatment option for many conditions and symptoms that are associated with PEIs, including certain headache syndromes such as cluster headaches and obstructive sleep apnea. Oxygen has a well-documented therapeutic effect on brain tissue.[2] Indeed, when any patient experiences focal or global ischemia (lack of blood flow)—for example, due to vasculitis or stroke, both of which are connected to Long Covid and other PEIs—we often induce hypothermia (a cold state) because it has neuroprotective abilities by lowering the metabolism of cerebral oxygen, thus rendering the ischemic tissue less needy for oxygen while slowing the rate of degradation of the oxygen molecules. I recommend some form of oxygen therapy to pretty much all of my patients, and I have three methods that I suggest.

Oxygen Concentrator

These are simply oxygen tanks like ones you've seen many times before, and they're the simplest, easiest, and most cost-effective method of oxygen therapy. The oxygen is usually administered in some dosage by way of a nasal cannula, a lightweight tube with prongs that is inserted into the nostrils. But sometimes a higher flow is needed, in which case the patient is fitted with a non-rebreather mask that delivers higher concentrations of oxygen and does not allow outside air to be inhaled. The more oxygen you can deliver efficiently and purely, the greater the

---

2 Cameron Rink and Savita Khanna, "Significance of Brain Tissue Oxygenation and the Arachidonic Acid Cascade in Stroke," *Antioxid Redox Signal* 14, no. 10 (May 2011): 1889–1903, https://www.ncbi.nlm.nih.gov/pmc/articles/PMC3078506/.

chance that the oxygen will find its way to the red blood cells to be picked up and carried. I typically have patients do two or three sessions per day of about thirty minutes each with two to four liters of oxygen.

The benefits of oxygen are so great, so widespread. I had a patient named Sarah who had chronic fatigue syndrome and the connective tissue disorder Ehlers-Danlos syndrome and a wide range of debilitating symptoms, but in her mind the biggest issue was sleep. She could not sleep, and that was all she wanted to talk about when she came to visit. She could fall asleep, but she never slept more than an hour or two at a time, and she was exhausted. Even when she did sleep, she was not waking up refreshed. She was in her early thirties, and I worked with her a long time. Eventually she was doing much better, but then the sleep issues started up again. I put her on a regular schedule of oxygen—thirty minutes in the morning, thirty minutes in the middle of the day, and then forty-five minutes right before bedtime. And almost right away she found that she would sleep four hours at a time, which was a huge improvement. Over time, as she continued using the oxygen consistently, her sleep got better and better to the point that she was sleeping most of the night and then all of the night. More important, she woke up feeling refreshed, which had not happened for her in years because she had chronic fatigue syndrome, and those patients never wake up feeling refreshed, even when they're sleeping eight hours a night. She also reported better cognitive function.

Many medical insurance companies will cover oxygen

concentrators with the right appeal information, even if you don't have a respiratory illness diagnosis. The recommended use is two to five liters per nasal cannula or oxygen headset (if nasal cannula is not tolerated) for twenty to thirty minutes up to three times daily as needed.

Hyperbaric Oxygen Treatment (HBOT)

Hyperbaric oxygen treatment is a highly touted therapeutic use of oxygen.[3] It involves going inside a special space called a hyperbaric chamber, in which the air pressure is raised to a higher than normal level, which helps the lungs take in greater quantities of oxygen. Not only are you adding oxygen molecules to your bloodstream, but with the increased pressure, or force, oxygen molecules have a better chance of perfusing or entering into the tissue or into the cells.

The positive effects of HBOT are well researched and well documented. Conventionally, it is used for wound healing, decompression sickness, and carbon monoxide poisoning, but its neuroprotective effects are becoming increasingly clear. We see benefits for various neurological disorders, including stroke, vasculitis, and, importantly, traumatic brain injury, which is especially relevant because

---

3 Fahimeh Ahmadi and Ali Reza Khalatbary, "A Review on the Neuroprotective Effects of Hyperbaric Oxygen Therapy," *Medical Gas Research* 11, no. 2 (April–June 2021): 72–82, https://www.ncbi.nlm.nih.gov/pmc/articles/PMC8130666/.

I see post-exposure illness as a form of brain injury. You have neuroinflammation, which is what a brain injury is, so you can benefit greatly from hyperbaric oxygen. The extra breathing force improves the movement of oxygen and the overall circulation of blood through both the medium and small vessels. It also helps to repair damaged tissue, reduces inflammation, and can even help reduce swelling of the brain.

HBOT is also very effective for connective tissue disorders. The reason it is used for wound healing is because it allows for proper collagen laydown and closure of disintegrated skin, and skin is made of connective tissue. It's got collagen in it. I already talked about how hyperbaric oxygen helps to support the reduction of inflammation, and when it reduces inflammation of the connective tissue, that allows for better structural alignment and better immune function, because the connective tissue actually has a lot of immune activity and function.

Not too long ago, I had a patient who was a graduate student at an Ivy League university and had Ehlers-Danlos syndrome, the connective tissue disorder, as well as many of the typical symptoms of post-exposure illness, particularly brain fog and a general inability to focus. It had gotten so bad for her that she had dropped out of her graduate program for a semester because she had so much trouble focusing on her studies. Reading was a particular challenge and, as with so many of my patients (and with you, perhaps), she felt like she had lost a part of who she was. She was an academic, but now she could not study or read. I worked with her in all the ways that I do, including prescribing medications and activity, and I suggested hyperbaric oxygen. As expected, the results she felt from the oxygen were remarkable—she felt much of that clarity and focus that had been missing, and the more times she did a session, the better it got. She felt so good when she was in the chamber that she started bringing her books to read in there.

Although HBOT is very effective, it takes some time. For the cumulative effect to be appreciated, patients usually need to undergo forty to sixty sessions, which could be weekly or even up to four or five times per week, for forty to sixty minutes per session. But if you are experiencing cognitive slowing, brain fog, or lightheadedness, it will likely be worth the effort, because HBOT is typically very effective for those symptoms.

Besides taking some time, the only other downside is that insurance will only cover it if you have severe wounds, like a burn patient, for example, despite the research supporting its therapeutic benefits for traumatic brain injury and neuroinflammation. So it is usually paid for out of pocket, and you have to go to a place that has hyperbaric oxygen chambers or tents. Do an internet search for clinics or centers near you that have HBOT machines for patient use. You will likely need a prescription to go to an HBOT clinic, which most doctors seeing you for your chronic symptoms should readily provide, and while I don't think these clinics are widely available yet, they are becoming more accessible every year. You may even be able to rent an HBOT tent so you can do the treatment at home, which is preferable because this therapy requires many sessions over many weeks.

Vasper

Admittedly, this treatment is pretty next-level because it's expensive and hard to find, and certainly if you're bed-bound or housebound you're not going to be able to use it right now. But I believe strongly in it, so I think it's important to share. If you get to a point where you're strong enough to go out, and you can find a Vasper clinic, it's an amazing way to increase the rate of your recovery.

Vasper is a sort of exercise bicycle that combines oxygen, compression, and hypothermia to compound the effects of the workout. You ride a reclined stationary bike while wearing an oxygen mask and cuffs around your thighs and arms, with your feet on freezing-cold brass plates. When you start to exercise, the cuffs are infused with ice-cold water, and you work out for twenty-one minutes doing a series of sprints and rests. Because of the cuffs, your blood flow is restricted during the exercise, and because of the hypothermia, your blood vessels are dilated much wider than usual. When the compression is released, there's a great rush of blood, almost an explosion of blood blasting through your wide-open veins, and that force pushes the blood into the muscles and into the brain. And because of the oxygen mask, that blood is infused with extra oxygen, so you're getting more oxygen and you're using it more efficiently. The effects are frankly astonishing, and they are completely sustained.

As I said, Vasper is not accessible for everyone, but some cities do have Vasper clinics, particularly in California. I sometimes have patients simulate the experience the best they can by putting towels in the freezer and then wrapping their thighs for a workout. Any cold exposure is therapeutic, by the way, including cold showers. You can take a regular hot shower and then, for the final twenty seconds, turn it to full-on cold to increase oxygen flow through the vessels and ease your sympathetic nervous system, which is in overdrive because of your symptoms. Cold showers may not sound pleasant, but I promise you will feel better afterward.

The Best Therapy of All: Get Outside

WHEN I WAS WORKING AS a contract researcher at the EPA for my dissertation on pharmaceutical residues in the environment, I was tapped by the program for Urban Landscape Design based in Durham, North Carolina, to help guide their goal to design green spaces within urban and city environments and to discuss the importance of access to green spaces for the health of the population at large. There is quite a bit of robust and dynamic research over the past few decades that has definitively proven the vast physical and mental benefits of exposure to nature.[4] Yet we are spending more and more time indoors instead of less. We sit in our homes, our cars, our offices, in restaurants, and more. We watch more TV, spend more time on our phones, computers, and tablets, and we spend less time connecting—with other humans and with the great outdoors. All this time indoors is not in any way good for our long-term health.

In fact, I would argue that it puts us at greater risk of developing chronic and complex illness and reduces our natural abilities for prevention and resilience. The outdoors offers us life. Going outside is like an infusion of what life is meant to be for humans. We evolved outdoors. We have innate desires for the benefits of the outdoors, but also the risks. "Fight or flight" is not just a catchphrase. It is a real, albeit simplistic, description of how our autonomic nervous system was designed. When we moved from outdoors to indoors, much of that system went unused or was used inappropriately, which is what you see with post-exposure illness. Our innate mechanisms that were

---

4 Mathew P. White et al., "Spending at Least 120 Minutes a Week in Nature Is Associated with Good Health and Wellbeing," *Scientific Reports* 9, no. 7730 (June 2019): https://doi.org/10.1038/s41598-019-44097-3; Rachel M. Nejade, Daniel Grace, and Leigh R. Bowman, "What Is the Impact of Nature on Human Health? A Scoping Review of the Literature," *Journal of Global Health* 12 (December 2022): https://www.ncbi.nlm.nih.gov/pmc/articles/PMC9754067/; Jim Robbins, "Ecopsychology: How Immersion in Nature Benefits Your Health," Yale Environment 360, January 9, 2020, https://e360.yale.edu/features/ecopsychology-how-immersion-in-nature-benefits-your-health.

designed to protect us from a tragic end at the hands of vicious predators or cataclysmic events are now recruited to protect us from microscopic, systemic, relentlessly provoking physiologic assaults. And sometimes "relentlessly" is the key word. In the form of an overactive immune system, that fight-or-flight mechanism is powerful, and it can do some damage, as you have seen.[5]

Now, I'm sure we're all very happy not to be running from saber-toothed tigers every day or trying to stay warm through the winter in a cave. Shelter is important, of course. But the more modern devices such as smartphones and smart TVs we acquire, and the more we drift toward overconsumption through digital platforms, the less we leave our constructed, enclosed abodes. And that comes with a price. The air we breathe in our homes and offices and other structures has been tainted with aerosols, product residues, mold species, and more. We're making ourselves sick.

Thankfully, the solution is simple, and it's one that can help alleviate your chronic symptoms. The most effective and meditative way of bringing in more oxygen to your being, your brain, and your body is to get outside.

---

5 Not that there were no microscopic organisms to contend with in prehistoric times. Of course there were. But there were fewer pathogens that we were exposed to, and there were also fewer interventions available, such as medications, and we were at the mercy of how virulent or pathogenic that organism was, which often meant a quick demise and not a progressive, life-altering, chronic state of unwellness.

Benefits of Getting Out

When my daughter was a kindergartener at Waldorf School in Seattle, each day the class would walk to the woodlands for a two-hour play period. It did not matter if there was snow, rain, wind, or sun in the forecast. They had to have appropriate gear for any weather, and it was all stored there in the school in their cubbies. Each morning when we arrived, a chalkboard showed a drawn figure of a child and the right clothing—rain pants, boots, hat, and so on—and we would dress our child as directed. And off they went into the woods, where they climbed trees, played with balls and Frisbees, rolled down hills, dug in the dirt, and just ran around laughing and singing. The kids became nature experts, which was very cool, but an added bonus was that they were excited to learn their lessons when they returned to their desks. They were more engaged, took deeper naps, and were overall happier children that year.

Exposure to nature has been shown to have positive effects on metabolism, blood pressure, cardiovascular health, inflammation, pain, and mental health. I don't think there is anything that rivals what pure nature can do for us. It is completely free, without side effects, easily accessible for the most part, and comes with significant and varied health benefits.

The flora in the natural landscape take up the carbon dioxide we exhale, and in exchange they give us oxygen back. Taking a deep breath of oxygen within a natural setting is the better option than through a tube in your bed or a mask in a room or even in a chamber (which, as I've said, can be an alternative way when illness prevents us from getting outside). Atmospheric pressure in a natural setting is optimal for healthy oxygen exchange, and you usually get the dual and natural benefit of movement, because when we're in a natural setting we're usually doing something like walking or hiking, which forces blood movement to pick up those oxygen molecules and transport them to where they are needed the most. All this helps support healing and recovery.

Finally, being outdoors engages the mind and brain. We take in amazing sensory experiences from nature, and there is always something to learn from natural landscapes. The shape of a leaf, the behavior of a particular species of bird, the sounds of the variety of birds in any one area, and the rolling appearance of mountainsides that seem so close yet are so far away—these don't only increase pleasant feelings and reduce feelings of anger, anxiety, and fear. They also stimulate our cognitive function. Research has shown that being exposed to natural environments improves cognitive flexibility, working memory, and attentional control. (Exposure to urban environments is linked to attention deficits.)

Being outside also just makes us feel good. Studies show that it helps us feel more contented and happier. It helps us feel more connected, not only to nature but to our communities. Chronic illness leads many of us to feel isolated and disconnected, as I did after my surgery. Getting into nature combats those feelings, too. Getting outside in the morning also has the added benefit of contributing to the reset of the circadian rhythm and will, in time, improve sleep.

Taking a break from the fret and struggle of illness is worthy of your time. Studies show patients recover from surgery better and with fewer complications when there are trees outside their hospital windows. Years ago there was a push to add more trees surrounding hospitals so that more patients could enjoy this benefit, but that seems to have fallen by the wayside, probably because, unsurprisingly, it was deemed unfavorable to the bottom line of the hospital.

Increasing Your Outdoor Time

Some studies have suggested urban dwellers have much higher rates of mental health difficulties and chronic illness than those who live in more pastoral areas.[6] To be fair, there are many more variables that play a role, and access to care is greater in urban areas, which may help decrease the suffering of mental health concerns. Urban landscape architects help design cities with parks, so that those who live within the city limits, even those living in lower socioeconomic regions, can take their children to the park, take their dogs to the park, exercise in the park, or just go to the park and breathe. And that may

---

6 Jiayuan Xu et al., "Effects of Urban Living Environments on Mental Health in Adults," *Nature Medicine* 29 (2023): 1456–67, https://www.nature.com/articles/s41591-023-02365-w.

be all it takes. Go to the park and breathe. Go into your yard, if you have one, and breathe. Or just stand in the grass somewhere. Doing this consistently and regularly can really boost your mental and physical health.

Doing things that require more time outdoors is even better. Having a picnic, watching the sunset, reading a book or listening to a podcast under a tree, napping in a hammock, fishing, bird-watching, and going to a farmers' market are just a few ideas. Better yet, of course, is if you can introduce some movement and activity: nature hikes, bike rides, gardening, swimming in a local lake, playing catch, building a snowman, having a snowball fight, hunting for bugs, swinging on the swings, shooting baskets, playing disc golf, skipping rocks . . . you get the idea. Sometimes it's nice to remember what it was like to be a kid.

The obvious problem, when you are chronically sick, is that it can be very hard to go anywhere, much less a campground or a hiking trail, or do anything even slightly vigorous. The good news is that starting with just going outside is effective. Stepping outside your home in the morning for morning light and deep breaths of fresh air each day can have positive cumulative health effects for most, if not all, organ systems. Walking down your street or your road allows for movement of blood to the lungs, heart, muscles, joints, and brain. And again, walking with a focus on your breath, inhaling through your nose and exhaling through your mouth, can also improve flow of cerebrospinal fluid. Increase your time outside and the vigor of your activities as you are able. You might be surprised how quickly you can build up your tolerance.

When I was recovering from brain surgery, there is no question the long walks in the woods that I regularly went on with a friend, or with my husband or my dogs, were critical to my healing journey. I was slow at first—almost embarrassingly so—but picked up speed and elevation with time. I focused on my breathing and how I felt with each step and each breath. Walking also helped distract me from my fears about my future and my health, and allowed me some mental clarity to plan. I was able to get a steady dose of vitamin D from the sun and improve my vagal tone (parasympathetic, or "rest and digest," function) from the chill. Every season had something to offer, and I always made sure I was wearing the appropriate attire. With my busy days now, I still take walks and get outside as much as possible, but I don't have as much time to spend just focusing on myself the way I did then. Even though those were very difficult days, I really miss those long walks in the woods.

Take-Home Guidelines

1. Oxygen is life! Breathing is key not only to our basic survival—being deliberate about our breathing can actually help us heal.
2. The fatigue, inactivity, and generally lousy feelings associated with chronic illness can lead us to breathe more shallowly, which impairs our recovery.

3. It might be worth trying oxygen therapy if it is available to you.
4. It is *definitely* worth getting outside consistently and frequently. Outside air is more healing than indoor air, and being outside naturally helps us be more active, too.

8

Sleep and Your Circadian Cycle

READ THIS CHAPTER TO FIND OUT . . .

- How sleep helps you heal, and how healing helps you sleep
- The critical role of your twenty-four-hour circadian cycle
- How to jump-start recovery through a healthy daily rhythm
- The relationship between trauma, stress, and sleep—and what you need to do about it

WE ALL KNOW HOW IMPORTANT sleep is. You probably know on an intellectual level that sleep is key to our mental and physical well-being, contributing to the health of every function and process in our bodies, and that good sleep is critical to good overall health while poor sleep vastly increases our risk for disease and other problems. More saliently, you know that you feel lousy when you don't get enough sleep, and you feel better when you do.

But let's sink deeper into sleep. (Sounds great, right?) I have no doubt that poor sleep is playing a major role in exacerbating your chronic symptoms, and in turn your chronic symptoms are making it harder to sleep. But there is plenty you can do to disrupt this cycle.

How Sleep Restores Us

IMAGINE YOUR SLEEPING BODY AS a hive of activity, where your nervous system is working hard to take care of you. Your brain is storing new information and creating memories and learning, and by way of the glymphatic system, which is like the waste management department of the brain, it is also getting rid of metabolic waste by-products and cellular debris from the many chemical reactions that take place within us all day. The glymphatic system also helps to remove abnormal proteins that form as a result of inflammatory processes in the brain. If these proteins are not removed, they accumulate in the brain tissue, where their presence has been linked to some forms of neurodegenerative diseases, including Alzheimer's disease. And the glymphatic system does even more for us. It also supports brain cellular renewal as well as the synthesis and metabolism of critical hormones and other compounds—such as dopamine, serotonin, glutamate, GABA, norepinephrine, histamine, and more—that we need in order to function and feel good during the waking activities of our daily lives. The waste of these activities is then taken out with the rest of the trash while we sleep.

The glymphatic system does all that waste management and caretaking for us, but here's the thing: It is primarily active while we sleep.

Sleep is also when we have uninterrupted production of cerebrospinal fluid, which not only lubricates and bathes the brain and spinal cord but aids the glymphatic system in doing its work of clearing the brain of toxic waste. CSF is also important for delivery of nutrients and substrates for all the functions of the brain such as memory, focus, attention, and immune surveillance. During sleep, neurons and other highly active brain cells recoup their own energy and rejuvenate because they are finally able to receive a steady supply of oxygen and cofactors that are not diverted for some activity that may occur during the day. They have their own dedicated stream of components they need for their own restoration.

Also active during sleep is your neuroendocrine system, a complex regulatory mechanism that includes the hypothalamus and the pituitary. The neuroendocrine system secretes five distinct hormones that are essential for many things, including metabolism, so if you feel sluggish instead of energized in the morning or throughout the day, it is probably because your hormone secretion during sleep is out of whack. These hormones also are critical to your healthy response to stress and your immune system. That's why good sleep is the elixir for most things.

It's also why our brains and our bodies are at their most vulnerable when we do not sleep, or do not sleep well. If our glymphatic system does not have time to take out the toxic trash and repair brain cells, if we're not producing enough CSF to help with waste removal and to deliver nutrients to the brain, and if our neuroendocrine system's secretion of essential hormones is disrupted—it's easy to see why our bodies would be compromised in their ability to withstand the assault of toxins and other foreign substances from the environment, or to bounce back from the degradation that happens within us due to chronic symptoms. So clearly, all these important physiologic changes that take place during sleep are intricately related to how well someone with a chronic illness can respond to treatment, and even to how much recovery you can expect. The effect of poor sleep has been well established and has been named its own risk factor for a number of diseases, including dementia syndromes, strokes, headaches, Parkinson's disease, immunocompromised states, and more.

Of course, for those with chronic and complex illness, this becomes something of a chicken-and-egg story because chronic illness can alter sleep function. Many of my patients report difficulty falling asleep or staying asleep, or waking several times throughout the night. Interestingly, when I dig a little deeper with them, many report a long history of sleep difficulty that preceded their illness. Sleep and disease and health are intimately interconnected. I had a patient not long ago, Maura, who was a video editor but had been on disability for some time when she came to me due to her chronic symptoms. She had not been sleeping well for years, so much so that it wasn't clear to her which came first, the sleep issues or the other symptoms. But it was the lack of sleep that she believed was affecting her life the most dramatically—and it was affecting every part of her life, not just her job. Perhaps most noticeably, it was taking a toll on her relationship with her wife, Linnea, who also was not sleeping because of Maura's restlessness. Maura and Linnea had planned to have children, but they had put their plans on pause due to Maura's illness, and as the weeks and months went by, this pause was creating more and more tension between them—Linnea was patient and understanding, but, as she said, neither of them was getting any younger. Linnea joined Maura for many of her visits with me, and when they talked about starting a family, they both cried as they held hands in my office, dark rings beneath their eyes. Maura's primary care doctor had prescribed several different medications, including Ambien and other sleep medications, antidepressants, even benzodiazepines. But nothing helped, and she and her wife both felt hopeless. She was struggling so much with sleep, and worrying about it so much, that she was not even addressing her other symptoms, which were also bad.

This is why sleep is a critical component for treatment of chronic illness, because when we don't sleep, not only is healing more of an uphill battle, but so is our ability to tolerate and adapt to our symptoms. Our functionality significantly decreases, as does our motivation to follow guidance from doctors and actively participate in our recovery, which impairs our chances of recovery and negatively impacts the therapeutic relationship with the doctor.

But It's Not Just Sleep

AS I HAVE SAID, MOST of us are quite aware of the importance of sleep, even if we don't fully understand all the reasons *why* it's so important. And for many of us, it is a struggle. As a society we spend huge amounts of money on sleep supplements and sleep medications, we use sleep apps to help calm our minds and bodies, we turn on noise machines and fans, all to help us fall into slumber. But sleep is only one part of the sleep-wake cycle of our days, and while zeroing in on sleep in these ways can be helpful, we do much better when we focus on our circadian rhythm as a whole, which means fixing our waking component as well as our sleep component.

We are circadian beings, which means our brains and bodies are meant to function on a cyclical rhythm. Basically, when it's light we are meant to be awake, and when it's dark we are meant to be asleep, because certain physiological things take place in our bodies and brains during those times. Obviously, in our modern world it's impossible to adhere to a strict light-and-dark routine. Where I live, in Seattle, the summer days are light until eleven P.M., and it is dawn at four A.M., and in winter it's just the opposite. I can't just sleep from eleven to four—that's not enough. Wherever you live, the length of the day changes throughout the year, and you have responsibilities that require you to do things at various times during the light and dark periods of the day, and so on. Most of this we can't control, but none of it changes the fact that every cell in our body has a certain circadian clock. Hormones and neurotransmitters are meant to be secreted in rhythms, some diurnal (during the day, such as cortisol) and some nocturnal (during the night, such as growth hormone, which is needed for rebuilding of tissues), and the rhythm of their synthesis and secretion can be altered when our sleep-wake rhythm is altered. For example, if you're getting up too early or late or at variable times, your adrenal glands won't know how much or when to pump out cortisol to get you going. If your cortisol levels are all over the place, then your pituitary and your hypothalamus are receiving confusing messages and in turn randomly producing adrenocorticotropic hormone (ACTH), which is meant to push the adrenal glands to make more cortisol, and that can lead to a feedback loop where hormonal levels are out of whack all day. And what happens when your hormonal levels are out of whack? You guessed it. You feel sluggish and lethargic. It's hard to get up in the morning, you don't feel focused, you have a hard time getting going and concentrating. You don't want to work that day, you don't want to engage in conversation, and you're not getting stuff done or feeling refreshed. You feel brain fog, which is one of the most common symptoms of chronic illness. In fact, low hormone levels, particularly cortisol and serotonin, are common among Long Covid patients, chronic fatigue syndrome patients, and other chronically ill populations.

The answer is to establish a twenty-four-hour routine and stick to it. Wake up at the same time each day. Have all your meals at the same time. Do your exercise at the same time. Do your meditation, if you do it, at the same time. Establish a bedtime routine where you start to wind down, go through the same rituals, and go to bed at the same time every day.

We instinctively do this with babies, right? We understand that they thrive on a schedule, and new parents strategize and coordinate so that their baby can follow a sleep, feed, and nap schedule. That routine allows their nervous systems to develop optimally, as they are in a constant state of neurodevelopment. While we, as adults, obviously cannot compete with the pace and activity of neuroplasticity and developmental stages of newborns, infants, and toddlers, we are nevertheless always in a state of the struggle between degeneration and regeneration, and even more so when we have been chronically exposed and chronically ill. A routine can help us. Unfortunately, over the years, we very easily and very quickly lose a routine that respects us as circadian beings. As we age, there seem to be more and more reasons why we abandon those routines, be it work, family, social activities, travel, stress, vices, or sickness. The lack of routine will eventually catch up with us and create not only sleep dysfunction but day-time dysfunction as well, with emotional disturbances, poor tolerance to pain, sleepiness, restlessness, fatigue, and more. Lack of routine may also cause structural, cellular, and metabolic changes to the brain. Indeed, screwed-up sleep stage cycling has been shown to cause changes in the expression of genes as well as epigenetic modifications that result in alteration of immune and inflammatory responses. For those who are chronically ill, this can further impede healing and recovery and worsen the course of disease.

It is particularly important to go to sleep and wake up at the same time each twenty-four-hour period. The first ninety-minute sleep cycle is the most beneficial with regard to secretion of growth hormone, initiation of the glymphatic system, and consolidation of memories and experiences from the day. This cycle should preferably take place between ten and eleven-thirty P.M., as studies have shown that for those who go to bed later, and their first cycle is at a later time in the night, that first cycle is less effective.

With chronic illness, it's even easier to stray off our natural rhythms, largely because we cannot do our usual activities, we don't feel well, cannot eat well, and may be at the mercy of scheduled appointments and caregivers whom we rely on to help us complete our needed tasks. I urge you to do what you can, because even small steps toward more of a routine can help us in exponential ways.

A Twenty-Four-Hour Schedule to Support Recovery

MY RECOMMENDATIONS FOR CORRECTING AND optimizing the sleep-wake rhythm are as follows. This is an idealized list—something to shoot for—and I realize that if you are struggling with chronic illness symptoms, and especially if your circadian rhythm has been in a state of disruption for a long time, this may seem futile. Many of my patients find it difficult to accomplish this entire list initially. But I believe it is important to begin in some fashion so that over time you can make small improvements, and even small improvements will allow for healing. The goal is to train the body and the brain back toward their internal clock. Do as much here as you think you can, and look to build on that over time.

Evening Fast

Do not eat during the three hours before bedtime. While we sleep, it is important that blood is sent to the organs that need to restore and regenerate. But if blood is being diverted to the gastrointestinal tract for digestion, metabolism, absorption, and assimilation, there is less blood supply that can go to the brain, nerves, and muscles. Not only that, but you're likely to experience suboptimal sleep because those gastrointestinal processes require a lot of energy, which also takes away from energy the body needs for restoration during sleep.

Evening Screen Fast

Discontinue all screens two hours before bed. Not only is the material you're consuming on screens likely to be stimulating, whether it's a movie or TV show or social media or even a book, but the blue light that screens emit tells our brains that it is time to be awake, forestalling its natural wind-down process. And it takes up time when you can be focusing on winding down. Many people like to read a (real) book instead of being on screens, and if that works for you, I say go for it. I love to read, but sometimes reading can energize me with ideas and interest, so I personally prefer puzzle books. Puzzles and games can be very relaxing, but remember to be doing them with pen and paper. A puzzle book with a pen or pencil may seem old school, but it has the desired effect.

Lavender Oils or Creams

Lavender is a great herbal nervine—it helps calm the nerves. I use lavender cream on my feet, focusing on important reflexology points for calm of mind and body, so I get the aromatherapeutic effects of the lavender as well as acupressure benefits. I also use a lavender mist for my sheets.

Reflexology Points on the Foot

There are many reflexology points on the foot and elsewhere around the body, and you can find body maps online to help guide you if you choose to do some acupressure on yourself. Meanwhile, here are the foot spots I like to focus on.

1. **The big toe:** The bottom of the big toe is believed to correspond to the head and neck area. Applying gentle pressure to this area may help relieve headaches or sinus congestion.

2. **The ball of the foot:** This area is associated with the chest and lung region. Stimulating this point may help with respiratory issues or feelings of tightness in the chest.

3. **The arch of the foot:** This area is connected to the digestive system. Massaging this point may aid digestion and relieve stomach discomfort.

4. **The heel:** This point is thought to be linked to the pelvic area. Applying pressure to this spot may be helpful for menstrual cramps or lower back pain.

5. **The inner edge of the foot:** This region is believed to correspond to the spine. Gentle pressure along this area may help alleviate back pain or tension in the back. From the heel/back of the foot up toward the toes simulates from the lumbar spine region up toward the cervical spine.

Consider Supplements

I often recommend melatonin, preferably in the form of dissolvable tablets because the veins on and beneath the tongue absorb at an appropriate rate to deliver it to the central nervous system. Melatonin is not a sleeping pill, so it does not necessarily work immediately, so I recommend taking it each night about thirty minutes before bed. Most people feel an improvement in their ability to fall asleep after doing this for about five days. It also seems to help smooth out the transition between sleep stages, which is when many people wake up due to jerky movements (referred to as myoclonus), and to decrease the number and frequency of headaches and migraines. Melatonin has also been shown to be mitoprotective, meaning it helps to support and protect the mitochondria. I generally do not recommend melatonin use for greater than three months at a time, so take a four- to six-week rest after three months, and you can go back to it after that if needed. Other supplements that can be helpful include magnesium, L-theanine, valerian root, and passionflower tincture. You can take these alongside melatonin or during your breaks from melatonin.

Quiet Time

Take fifteen minutes to sit quietly prior to getting into bed. You don't have to meditate, though that is preferred and should be your eventual goal. (When you do meditate, you can choose most any meditation app or exercise you find and like, and it does not have to be long. Shoot for just a minute or two at first.) But to start, just be still and quiet. Note your heart rate and your breath. Take deep breaths in and exhale deep breaths out. Try hard to focus on your breath. When a thought or a worry or even a vision comes to your mind, try to just watch it as it passes on through. Don't give it a single minute of your energy or attention. Wave bye to it for now.

Dark Room

It's important that the room is very dark. Hang blackout curtains and remove all devices that emit even the slightest light, including your phone, which should be charged in a separate room. The way we live these days rarely allows for complete darkness. In addition to screens, we have clocks and other appliances in our bedroom that have small lights that, even if minimal, nevertheless disrupt the darkness. We also must contend with the lights of our neighbors, the lights on our streets, and the overall light of the city in which we live. Even low-level light can penetrate the eyelid and disrupt sleep cycles. I used to live in Las Vegas, and it was never completely dark. Even where I live now, in Seattle, which by every standard is gray and gloomy in the winter, there are still many lights throughout the street. I wear an eye mask each night, which I highly recommend.

Cool Room

As discussed earlier, cold exposure stimulates the part of the nervous system that controls resting activity and opens your blood vessels to allow more blood to flow to parts of the body that need it, so it relaxes the body. There are many cold exposure therapy programs for health and wellness, but one thing you can easily do is keep your room cool when you go to bed. During summer months, I recommend even putting an ice pack in the bed next to your body. It should not touch the body but be close by, emanating its cold air. If you have the budget for it, there are some great mattresses with chill settings on the market.

Body Scan

When you first get into bed, do what I refer to as a body scan, starting with your toes and moving up your body. Connecting to each body part within your brain helps to relax your mind and your body. Close your eyes and connect your brain to your toes so that you feel their presence. Do not move them, or any body part as you connect with it. After focusing on your toes for a few seconds, connect with your calves in the same way. Then move on to your knees, thighs, hips, abdomen, lungs, heart, fingers, arms, shoulders, lips, nose, cheeks, eyes, ears, and head. You can also do it when you wake during the night and have difficulty falling back to sleep. This is a self-directed relaxation technique that can greatly calm a wired brain.

Supported Positioning

Chronic illness from chronic exposures is damaging to the connective tissue, so it is important to support your body's alignment as much as possible when sleeping so you do not wake up with a kink, which can result in dislocation, subluxation, or injury. If it is in your budget, you can make sure your back and neck are supported with one of the many ergonomic pillow options available on the market. Appropriate ergonomics also includes a slight elevation of your head and neck, which aids circulation from the glymphatic system, cerebrospinal fluid, and blood supply vasculature. Importantly, supporting only your head with just a pillow can sometimes flare symptoms related to craniocervical instability as it further "folds" that upper cervical region contributing to the compression, making the alignment worse, and, because we are sleeping, can result in tight and painful neck and scalp muscles.

Slow Start

When you awaken in the morning, stand slowly from bed to avoid muscle injury and to decrease your risk of light-headedness, dizziness, or hypoperfusion (disturbance in mental equilibrium brought on by sudden reduced blood flow and thus reduced oxygen and nutrients reaching the brain tissue). I recommend sitting on the side of the bed with your feet on the floor and waiting as you get your bearings and feel steady enough to stand slowly. It is an interesting phenomenon that strokes and heart attacks often occur in the morning upon awakening.

Water Detox

As part of your morning routine, drink a large glass of room-temperature water to aid excretion from the physiological events during the night. You can add lemon for extra digestive action and some taste, as well as a pinch of salt.

Morning Light Exposure

Go outside for at least twenty minutes to get exposure to morning light between the hours of six A.M. and ten A.M. This is a way for the brain to receive the morning light as a signal that this is a new day. The angle of the sun during different times of the day is perceived differently by the eyes, which then relay messages to the brain—specifically the hypothalamus and the reticular activating system, the areas where sleep and wake cycles are regulated. You can go for a walk or just sit outside. It does not have to be active and incorporate any movement, but it does need to be outside; sitting in the window won't do the trick because the light is diffused by the glass. While outside, take intentional deep breaths to get the lungs and heart moving and promote the circulation and delivery of oxygen and removal of carbon dioxide.

Schedule

During your day, try to schedule meals and movement at around the same time each day. Aim to be in bed approximately the same time each night and to wake approximately the same time each morning. It will likely be almost impossible initially, but this is all about the long game. None of what I'm suggesting here is a medicine or a cure, and your sleep is not going to be totally improved—or even perceptively improved at all—at first. But as I have said, it's important to start somewhere, and the hope is that over time your own natural rhythm will be awakened.

That's what happened with Maura, my patient who had put off having children with her partner, Linnea. I had asked her to keep a journal about her daily routine, and when I read it, it was clear that she did not have much of a daily schedule at all, except for one thing: Linnea came home from work after eight P.M. each night, and the two of them usually ate dinner together after that, which was way too late to be eating. So the first thing I told Maura was that she had to eat no later than six. I know it's nice to eat with your spouse or family, but eating so late was too disruptive to her sleep. And then we began to work on her schedule for the full day, starting with the morning. We established a set time for her to wake up every day, and when she woke up she slowly sat and then stood. She drank a glass of water and went outside to get morning light. While there, she did some breathing exercises and gentle stretches. She took the dog for a short walk twice a day, which she did on a schedule. She reserved a certain time in the afternoon for household chores or light exercise, and she ate her meals at the same time each day, including dinner at five-thirty. When Linnea came home, Maura would sit with her at the table and have a glass of water while Linnea ate. For bedtime, I prescribed a routine that began with a cup of chamomile tea with valerian tincture in it, which she drank about an hour before bed. About half an hour before bed she took melatonin (which, honestly, I was shocked she had not tried yet, as it has become pretty mainstream), and then she took a warm shower where she turned the water to 100 percent cold for the final twenty seconds. Maura was concerned that the cold shower would actually awaken her before bed, but she did it anyway, and she found that after getting out and toweling off, she was very relaxed—more so than she was after just a warm shower. Finally, I gave her a meditation exercise to do before bed, and eventually she even added blackout curtains to the bedroom to ensure that it was as dark as possible. She did not notice a change in the first week, but within a month's time she was sleeping remarkably well, and so was Linnea, whose sleep had been disrupted by Maura's restlessness. By the time Maura was winding down her visits with me, the two of them were talking again about starting their family.

I WANT TO SAY AGAIN that I know this can be hard. There are a lot of things that are just an ingrained part of living in our modern society that make it hard to be on a regular schedule and that keep us from being active, which is what makes us tired enough to sleep. We spend a lot of time sitting in our cars and in our offices, in front of the TV, looking at our phones and computers, and it's hard to break these habits. Some of it we can't break. We can't quit our jobs. But we were meant to be searching, exploring, and gathering during the day, moving, exerting muscular energy, thinking about ways to avoid predators and where to go to find the most nutritious berries. Moment-to-moment life used to require a lot of work from us physically and cognitively, and for the most part life is not like that anymore. It is no wonder we have insomnia. Even if we do get on a good schedule, sometimes we have a bad day—we're not very active that day, or we eat poorly or we eat late, or we eat inflammatory foods or drink alcohol. And for those who are chronically ill, it's easy to fall into a spiraling state of sadness about our loss of functionality in our lives, and that too can make it harder to do the things we need to do to stay on a schedule and start getting better. We feel lousy, and we graze all afternoon, and we watch YouTube videos, and before we know it, it is eleven o'clock at night and we're trying to go to sleep, and that just does not work.

Please remember: Every day is another opportunity to get back on schedule. Every day is another chance to take at least one small step toward recovery. No matter your situation, everyone can get outside for twenty minutes in the morning. You may not be able to do all the things on the list and keep a perfect schedule, but you need to at least focus on the things that you can control, because that will only help. It will absolutely not make things worse.

Dealing with Migraines When Traveling

Many of my patients suffer from headaches and migraines, which are hard enough to deal with when you're at home. But when you're traveling, it becomes a lot more difficult, not least because your sleep schedule and routine are disrupted. Sleep deprivation and fragmentation can easily cause migraines. Patients have frequently asked me how to deal with headaches and migraines when traveling, and even when not traveling. If migraines are a problem for you, here are a few tips.

1. To give yourself the best chance of getting good sleep, be sure to pack the things you need to ensure it. That may include melatonin, tea, tinctures such as valerian and ashwagandha, and your favorite pillow. Using an app for white noise or meditative music can be very helpful. Change of time zones can be problematic, so work to mimic your usual sleep routine and circadian rhythm as best you can.

2. Make sure you stay hydrated. Start each day with a large glass of water and a little salt to help keep your brain and body hydrated.

3. Maintain your usual food plan as best as possible. Avoid known food triggers, which can sometimes be a challenge when traveling. Try not to stray from foods you know work well for you. Avoid increased sugar, dairy, and fermented or processed food. Minimize alcohol and avoid wine.

4. Be active. Walk, bike, hike as much as you can. Get outdoors. Take deep breaths in nature. All have been

shown to lessen anxiety and fears, and improve blood flow to the brain.

5. Cold exposure can induce a parasympathetic ("rest and digest") state. Turn the water to cold at the end of your shower for ten seconds.

6. Try to schedule a massage (or two!) during your travels to help relax muscles and reduce anxiety over getting a migraine.

7. If traveling where there is plenty of sun, wear sunglasses (and sunscreen!). Be aware that direct bright light can be a migraine trigger.

8. Pack your daily preventative medications and be sure to be compliant about taking them.

9. Pack your abortive medications and always have them on you. Have a lower threshold to take them if you feel a migraine starting. You can use over-the-counter analgesics (ibuprofen, acetaminophen) and anti-inflammatories if need be when you feel a migraine starting.

10. Pack your migraine-targeted supplements, including magnesium, quercetin, and B complex. Be sure to take them each day.

Correct Anything That Is Disrupting Sleep

WHILE I DO EMPHASIZE THE importance of establishing a healthy and consistent twenty-four-hour cycle, it's also true that you need to correct anything that is directly interrupting sleep. So if you have sleep apnea, for example, you need to fix it, because it's important not to spend your nights in a state of low oxygen. And the only way to find out if you have something disrupting sleep is with a sleep study, which I highly recommend that you get. Fortunately, sleep studies can now be done at home; it is no longer necessary to spend nights in sleep centers, which used to be its own barrier for a truly reliable sleep study.

Besides sleep apnea, a sleep study can also identify abnormal heart rate, blood pressure, respiratory rate, and even muscle movements. It also offers valuable information on transitions between sleep stages and how long you spend in each stage, or even if you get to all the stages. The insight into what is happening to your brain while you are sleeping, or at least trying to, can be useful for any physician working with chronic illness, so let your doctor know when you get a sleep study and share the results with them. They may prescribe or recommend any of a number of fixes for any sleep dysfunction you have, including a CPAP machine. I have already talked about using oxygen before bed—sometimes the brain wakes up because it's not getting enough oxygen, and uploading oxygen before sleep is a good way to start out ahead of the game a little bit. If your brain is not getting enough oxygen during sleep, home oxygen is something I highly recommend. However you do it, you have to find ways of correcting things that are disrupting sleep because if you don't do that, trying to correct your twenty-four-hour cycle—and all of the circadian rhythmic release of hormones and neurotransmitters that are critical for healing mechanisms for the body to return to a less inflamed state—will be an uphill battle. If your brain is not getting oxygen, it's going to constantly wake you up asking for oxygen.

Pharmacologic sleep aids can also be helpful, by the way, and I often prescribe them. Many of my patients prefer to avoid these medications for fear of addiction or at least reliance, and maybe you feel similarly, which I totally understand, but there really is a benefit to using them for the short term if not longer. Pharmaceuticals can help us make progress faster than natural approaches alone. The use of sleep medications can remind your body and brain just what it feels like to sleep, what it feels like to fall asleep at a more natural hour, and what it feels like to stay asleep for more than a few hours. And if accompanied by natural approaches to correct the circadian disruption, over time, you will experience an even more beneficial effect. There are several sleep aids available over the counter, but if they are not working for you, my preferred pharmacological sleep aids include gabapentin, nortriptyline, low-dose naltrexone, mirtazapine, trazodone, and eszopiclone. Most of these have additional benefits for the symptoms of chronic and complex illness including decreased pain, improved mast cell reactivity, and mood stabilization.

Bottom line, if you're struggling with sleep, get a sleep study. You can start by asking your primary care doctor to order it, or seek out a sleep specialist (who are either neurologists or pulmonologists) on your own. It's often covered by insurance, and as I said, it can be done at home these days. And talk to your doctor about starting on a sleep aid. Solid, restorative sleep is just too important to mess around with. Get it fixed.

Addressing Trauma and Stress

IT'S VERY HARD TO FIND the peace of mind and body needed for optimal sleep, not to mention for healing, if we have trauma that has not been processed. Our cells hold memory, as the saying goes, and traumatic events cause a change in the expression of our genome and ultimately a change in protein synthesis and degradation, all of which changes cellular machinery, signaling, and functioning. In other words, trauma makes our cells less resilient. Our trauma, when unprocessed, continues to hurt us. And let's be clear: If you have been dealing with chronic complex illness for any length of time, that is traumatic. There is so much you may have lost, from mobility to your love of life to family and friends, perhaps a job. You may have been highly functional before this, and losing that is traumatic. Once you are better, you will have PTSD from this. You're going to have to work on this trauma.

You may also have had trauma before this. I have had patients who have had horrible trauma. So whether you've had earlier trauma or only trauma related to your chronic illness, that trauma has to be processed as part of the recovery, because it's going to be hard for the cells to be receptive to all that we're doing if they're holding on to these traumatic experiences.

I mentioned getting help for PTSD after you're better, but you will get the most benefit if you start working on it to the extent that you can now. And this can be done through work with a licensed therapist, psychologist, or psychiatrist. There are many modalities that can be successfully used, and these include eye movement desensitization and reprocessing (EMDR), biofeedback, neuroplasticity programs, and even ketamine-assisted psychotherapy. This work will heal you, and in turn you will sleep better, and that in turn will heal you more. Psychedelics are proving to have important roles in trauma-related disorders, especially psilocybin.[1]

It is also important to manage stress in our lives so that our fears and anxieties do not come to the forefront just when we need to sleep. This happens because we are usually distracted during the day and don't really pay attention to, well, what is on our mind. One method for preventing stress from bubbling to the surface at bedtime is to designate a different time—preferably the same time each day—when you spend twenty to thirty minutes thinking through current stressors in your life, even if the main stressor is your illness. Writing them down or saying them out loud during this time helps you feel like

---

1 Amanda J. Khan, Ellen Bradley, Aoife O'Donovan, and Joshua Woolley, "Psilocybin for Trauma-Related Disorders," *Current Topics in Behavioral Neuroscience* 56 (2022): 319–32, https://pubmed.ncbi.nlm.nih.gov/35711024/.

you have addressed them, and they are less apt to flood your brain at night.

Again, this can start a healthy cycle wherein dealing with your stress and trauma helps you sleep better, and sleeping better helps you deal with your stress and trauma. There are physiological reasons why optimizing our sleep can help with stress and trauma. During sleep, our subconscious brain works to consolidate events that have happened to us, but there is also packaging and relocation of those memories away from the hippocampus—the primary memory center of our brain—to other parts of the brain. When events cannot be packaged and relocated due to poor sleep, it is believed that contributes to PTSD. Stress and trauma keep us sick. It has been shown that stress responses to events and happenings in our lives increase epinephrine. Epinephrine increases mast cell degranulation and impairs healing of all sorts of tissue damage, mainly of connective tissue. As you can see, there are real physical reasons why we need to work on how our bodies and brains receive, interpret, and modulate stressful times. That is why I strongly suggest that you find a therapist or other professional to help you deal with your trauma.

I also recommend Ayurvedic treatments, the traditional healing practices that originated in India thousands of years ago. Ayurveda is a holistic system of medicine that focuses on achieving balance and harmony in the body, mind, and spirit. Ayurvedic treatments involve a range of natural therapies, including herbal remedies, dietary adjustments, lifestyle modifications, meditation, and various forms of bodywork such as massage and yoga. These treatments are personalized to an individual's unique constitution, known as their dosha, which is determined by their physical and mental characteristics. Ayurvedic treatments aim to promote overall well-being, prevent illness, and restore health by addressing the underlying imbalances in the body. Shirodhara, in which medicated oils or other liquids are slowly and steadily dripped onto the forehead, is a favorite of mine, and my patients regularly report increased calm and relaxation with reduced anxiety after doing it. They even report improvements in their symptoms, especially during times of flares. Do an internet search to find an Ayurvedic treatment center near you. If you are able to seek Ayurvedic treatments regularly and consistently, you may gain cumulative improvements in symptoms and your state of inflammation.

Avoiding Stress

ONE FINAL THOUGHT ABOUT SLEEP, trauma, and stress: While it is critical to process trauma and manage stress, the goal is to try to engage on a consistent basis with positivity, hope, and optimism. Working with a therapist, externalizing your anxiety, and engaging in other therapies are all great ways to try to heal trauma and cope with stress, but it's just as important to try to avoid more stress, anxiety, and negative energy. And one reliable source of negative energy is the internet, specifically social media. Too often, I see patients devolve into a state of despair that is compounded by engaging in negative spaces and with negative people online.

There are clear benefits to social media groups for the chronically ill, mainly that a good group can be a support system that you may have lost when you became ill. The sad truth is that as much as they may want to be supportive, family members, friends, colleagues, and others may not know how to support you when you do not return to good health in what seems like a reasonable time, and, worse, many may not even believe you. One patient told me her own mother told her to "just get out of bed and go to work." This alone is not only heartbreaking but also traumatic. So social media groups can be a lifeline. Another benefit of social media groups is education, for sure. In fact, I often marvel at how educated my patients are, and to be honest I find it helps move our conversation at a more direct pace and fashion.

But sometimes being immersed in a group of people who suffer similarly can sap our hope and inaccurately confer a sense of futility for any chance of recovery. I believe in the power of the mind as just one spoke in the wheel of healing. We must believe there is a chance we can get well. We must embrace the physiologic and anatomic obstacles in front of us. That positive energy should be spread and embraced. It is what I try to imbue in my patients because I have seen improvements along the way.

Those improvements do not come easily, nor do they come quickly, but they do come.

So if you are using social media to communicate with others who have similar symptoms to you or who have the same diagnosis, be honest with yourself as to whether this is a positive experience. Are you getting more education or support, or is it pulling you down? When it comes to social media, not only is it a good idea to get off screens a couple hours before bedtime, but it might also be wise to take an extended break and seek out positive spaces elsewhere. Reach out to close friends, family, or your partner and have a talk. Listen to music that makes you feel good. Journaling, meditation, and humming are all reliable ways to inject positivity into our lives. Laughter is especially effective, even if it's forced, because it releases endorphins and straight up makes us feel good. You can always go back to social media. In the meantime, you might find that you sleep better without so many (hurting, demoralized) voices in your feed—a feed that, as many of us know, can follow us into the darkness at bedtime.

Take-Home Guidelines

1. Sleep restores us. It's not just rest, and it does not just feel better when we sleep—there are critical physiological processes that need to happen during sleep, and if we are not sleeping well, we cannot get better. Period.
2. You can't just fix your sleep, though. You must develop a healthy, consistent twenty-four-hour circa-

dian rhythm. Wake time and sleep time depend on each other.

3. Get a sleep study so you can address any sleep dysfunction.

4. Chronic complex illness is traumatic. Address your trauma with a licensed therapist or other professional. Deal with your stress, too.

9

Regenerative Therapies

READ THIS CHAPTER TO FIND OUT . . .

- How new advances in modern medicine have increased our body's natural ability to heal itself
- How regenerative therapies work and how they help
- Which therapies you can do on your own, and which you can pursue with a healthcare professional

SUSAN WAS A FORTY-EIGHT-YEAR-OLD SOCIAL worker with a connective tissue disorder related to Sjogren's syndrome, an autoimmune disease that wreaks havoc on the body's moisture-producing glands and sometimes its vital organs. She suffered terribly from pain in her joints and along her spine. First-line treatment for Sjogren's syndrome greatly helped many of her symptoms, including the classic dry eyes and dry mouth, as well as some of the skin rashes she suffered from, but it did not touch the pain, which was interfering with her ability to work and engage in social and family activities. It interfered with her sleep and her movement. We worked hard to design an anti-inflammatory diet, and she was diligent about following it, and while some days the pain seemed better, she often flared. That's when we decided it was time to try something else. She found a doctor to give her a shot of prolotherapy (a dextrose solution that helps rebuild collagen, among other things) in her neck, shoulders, and hips, and she reported an almost immediate reduction in the pain. We decided to continue with prolotherapy, and the pain continued to respond with subsequent injections.

One of the amazing things about the human body is its ability to heal itself in so many ways. We cut a finger slicing veggies, it will heal. We get a nasty kink in the neck (probably from staring down at our phones), it will get better with time. Maybe more time than we'd like, but it will happen. And of course, if we catch a virus such as strep throat or Covid-19, we will recover.

Unfortunately, our natural healing abilities have limits. Cancer, heart disease, diabetes, arthritis, Alzheimer's, cystic fibrosis, and Crohn's disease—as well as Long Covid, mast cell activation disorder, chronic fatigue syndrome, and other PEIs that we're talking about in this book—are all examples of chronic conditions that our body cannot fight on its own. What we can do is manage our symptoms with medications and therapies, and that can certainly offer us a lot of relief and recovery.

Recently, though, due to technological breakthroughs, a new kind of therapy is expanding on the body's ability to repair itself. Regenerative therapies are, as the name implies, ways of regenerating or rebuilding tissue, supporting the body's natural ability to repair and restore itself so that patients can experience fuller recovery. For people who have chronic illness that stems from an inflammatory attack that never ends, be it from infection, exposure, or toxicity from a medication that was prescribed, the cellular damage they experience ultimately results in cells that are lost. With regenerative therapies, we can halt that degeneration and loss and begin regeneration of damaged tissue that may have difficulty returning to a functioning state. As I often say to my patients: We have to stop the degeneration so we can start the regeneration. And that's what we do.

Peptide Therapies

REGENERATIVE THERAPIES COME IN MANY forms, including injections, IVs, oral medication, nasal sprays, topical creams—even electrical and light therapies—and some of them you can do on your own at home. I recommend beginning with peptide therapies, which hold great regenerative potential and are not used as commonly as they should be. Peptides are fragments of proteins made up of a sequence of amino acids, and they have the ability to stimulate cellular repair and regrowth. Our bodies naturally make peptides, and they can be found in every cell in the body. They also can be found in other plant and animal sources.

Peptides are easy for the body to absorb, and they work by incorporating themselves into the membrane layers of cells and improving the function of the activity of that membrane, thereby improving the outcome of the intended purpose of that cell. There is still a lot of research to be done to better understand the mechanism of action of peptides, but peptide therapies are showing great promise for the treatment of metabolic disorders, pain, inflammation, immune disorders, and more. Each peptide targets a different kind of tissue, so you can be very precise in terms of which peptides you use and what tissue you are aiming to regenerate.

There are many peptide options available, and you may be aware of peptides sold as dietary supplements in the form of shakes or pills. They claim to help you lose weight and build muscle, though there is little evidence to back up those claims. You can also get skin products with peptides in them, which can help repair your skin in various ways, though I would be skeptical about the viability of peptides in creams on a shelf. What we're talking about here, though, is peptides to be taken as medication.

By far the peptides I have found most effective for chronically sick patients are GHK-Cu and BPC157 for their ability to improve the structure of the collagen and the connective tissue that holds our musculoskeletal, neuromuscular, and neurovascular systems together. These peptides are anti-inflammatory and analgesic (pain-relieving), and they help lay down intact collagen fibers so the architecture is more stable. And, importantly, these peptides help reduce the formation of scar tissue. People with connective tissue dysfunction from chronic and unaddressed inflammation suffer persistent, perpetual breakdown of tissue that then tries to repair itself but does so waywardly, resulting in scarring. These peptides can help improve this breakdown and repair process.

GHK-Cu peptide—which stands for glycyl-L-histidyl-L-lysine-Cu(2+)—is a naturally occurring copper peptide that can be found in our blood, urine, and saliva. It has potent biological activity and has been used in conventional medicine for wound healing in cases of trauma and burns. This peptide also has anti-inflammatory and antioxidant properties, so it packs a powerful punch in the effort to reduce inflammation and protect from oxidative stress that comes from hyperinflammation. GHK-Cu has also been shown to induce apoptosis (programmed and methodical cell death) in cancer cells or other types of atypical cells that can interfere with a healing state—an added bonus.

BPC157 is made of fifteen amino acids that are also found in the human body. It too is anti-inflammatory and protects against oxidative damage, and it too can help repair connective tissue, including ligaments, tendons, and muscles. It also has been shown to improve chronic gastrointestinal distress as well as improve blood flow including to the brain, and has been used to treat traumatic brain injury, neuroinflammatory and degenerative states, and even post-stroke patients.

ARA290 is another peptide, eleven amino acids long, that helps repair innate immune activity and has been very helpful for patients with neuropathy, glucose dysregulation, and pain.

These peptides can be purchased online in different forms, but it is very important that you work with your doctor on this as there are many, many peptides, and an appropriate plan for your symptoms should come from a discussion between you and your doctor.

When You Talk to Your Doctor About . . .
Peptide Therapy

Tell your doctor that you're interested in trying peptide therapy, and you can mention ARA290, GHK-Cu, and BPC157 as possibilities, and mention the reasons why (which are discussed above). As of October of 2023, peptide therapies can no longer be prescribed by doctors, but they are available over the counter online, and your doctor can help you choose the appropriate peptides and dosage. You can ask your doctor to recommend an online vendor, or research sources on your own. Be diligent in identifying reputable vendors.

Stem Cell Therapy

INFECTIONS AND OTHER EXPOSURES THAT affect
the immune system and lead to perpetual immune response create damage to our cells—all our cells—except
for one kind, our stem cells. Our stem cells are not affected, because they are not yet differentiated enough into
the mature cells they are destined to be, which means they
don't yet have the appropriate proteins on their membrane
surface to recognize and receive the incoming assault from
the immune system. Stem cells are the body's raw materials, the cells from which all other specialized cells will
develop, and they are our A-team soldiers for when we are
losing the war with infection because they can be used to
generate healthy cells to replace damaged ones.

Stem cells are held and nurtured within protected areas, yet they are accessible. In adults they are located in
bone marrow and in fat. You have heard of bone marrow
transplants: They are actually stem cell transplants, which
is when a donor's stem cells replace a patient's cells that
have been damaged by disease or chemotherapy, or they
help the donor's immune system to fight some types of
cancer and blood-related diseases. But we can also have
our own stem cells harvested from the fat on our body, filtered, and put back into us through an IV or an injection,
which can be a very effective way to spur our body to make
even more stem cells, greatly aiding tissue regeneration.
Because stem cells contain DNA, our own stem cells can

potentially give us this benefit without introducing foreign genomic material. Once inside of us, they migrate to where there is acute inflammation or chronic damage by reading signals. The signals of inflamed or damaged cells are much "louder" than those of healthy cells, so the stem cells know where to go, stop, and develop. It can take months for new cells to differentiate so that there are enough to improve organ function—just as it takes nine months for a baby to develop in the womb—and so effects, while they can be profound, can take a while, and patients usually need more than one round of injection or infusion. This kind of stem cell therapy is growing in popularity.

But so is exosome therapy. Exosomes are extracellular vesicles that contain growth factors and other substrates necessary for regeneration and communication between cells. They work faster than stem cells because upon infusion they release anti-inflammatory mediators and growth factors right away, whereas stem cells have to figure out where to go and what cell to differentiate into. Upon impact, exosomes release these important mediators, and many people have seen a noticeable effect of improved pain, mobility, stability, and fatigue.

Exosomes do not contain DNA, and they cannot be harvested from the patient like stem cells can. But they do contain RNA, which is an expression of DNA and used to make the many proteins of our bodies. So exosome therapies contain RNA that is not the patient's own. It is important to understand this distinction. Exosomes are isolated from placental tissues by a few companies in the United States.

If any of this sounds scary or expensive or out of reach, I want to say something important here, which is that you do not need to undergo harvesting and/or IV infusions to mobilize your stem cell count. There are many strategies we can employ on our own to do just that. The very fact that we have stem cells in our bodies as adults means that the body is ready and able to help rejuvenate and repair. In fact, this is the stem cells' job, one of the only reasons they are there. They want to be able to repair and heal. We just have to help them along, and you can do that without any outside help or medicine, simply from how you live. One of the best ways to do that is by fasting. Fasting has been proven to increase stem cells as well as combat neurodegeneration, among other benefits, as discussed in Chapter 5. There are many other lifestyle things you can do to boost stem cells, things we have talked about in this book, such as keeping a regular circadian rhythm, using an infrared sauna, engaging in aerobic exercise, lifting heavy weights, reducing sugar intake, increasing restorative sleep, doing cold exposure, and getting into nature. All these strategies are proven to boost stem cells and therefore regenerate damaged tissue and help you recover. And while it takes a little more effort when one is suffering from chronic inflammation and chronic disease, every little bit can help.

This is what Susan, the social worker, did. Once the shots she was receiving reduced the pain enough for her to be more engaged in her recovery, we then embarked on intensive therapy to help her body enhance production of her own stem cells. She used an infrared sauna, she engaged in safe fasting protocols, did yoga positions with support, and continued her anti-inflammatory diet, adding in juicing with green vegetables. We then added cold exposure and HBOT, both of which are thought to mobilize stem cells, and over the next six months she noted decreased pain to the point that she was able to live her life again. It's incredible to think about, really, that we literally have the power to regenerate tissue through our own lifestyle decisions.

But it is hard work. Changing your diet is hard work. Exercising, changing your schedule—it is hard work, but you can empower yourself to do it. If you are willing to be uncomfortable for a little while, it will become less uncomfortable. It gets easier, and it's going to make you feel better in the long run. That's all it takes.

LET'S TALK ABOUT AGING

I've long believed that stem cells are the future of medicine. They have an incredible ability to regenerate tissue and to repair damaged organ tissue that has been dying off, including nerves and muscles. In fact, there has been a lot of good research showing how stem cells can have regenerative powers for people with MS, people with ALS, and people with Alzheimer's. It is amazing what they can do.

There's also been a lot of research into the effect of stem cells on aging, much of it coming out of the longevity movement. You may have heard of this movement. Basically, wealthy people are pouring tons of money into figuring out how to stay alive much longer than the average human lifespan and stay healthy as well. I'm fascinated by this world for many reasons, but I'm quite interested in their research in particular. I started to wonder if some of the things that the longevity people were doing would be helpful for my patients, and lo and behold, they are.

In a way, aging—the fact of it, the act of it, the resistance against it—is the primary narrative of our lives, right? But if you have a post-exposure illness, you are aging more rapidly than you otherwise would. And the reason is all that inflammation we have talked about. The term often used is "inflammaging." One way to look at aging is, it's basically the effects of inflammation, and as we get older our body's ability to suppress that inflammation wanes. Every decade of life we lose a little bit of reserve with regard to how resilient our body is. And of course, the burden of exposures increases as we live. Every decade, there's more that accumulates in our bodies.

The good news is that age does not seem to affect how well a patient responds to treatments for their PEI symptoms. So a patient in their sixties might be more susceptible to certain symptoms because their resilience is lower than a patient who is in their thirties. But the treatments I am talking about in this chapter and throughout this book have almost as much potential at being effective, no matter the decade of life.

Many of my patients travel to other countries to go to stem cell clinics, and I am clear with them that I do not keep up with the regulations in other countries and I can't vouch for the safety of any given clinic. But the information is out there to pursue this if you can afford it.

Stem cells can be remarkably effective, and while I used to be skeptical, and even fearful because they are not approved by the FDA for these indications, I can't argue with the benefits I have seen in my patients that have found places to get autologous stem cells.[1] I have noted decreased insulin requirements in my patients with diabetes, improved strength in my patients with mitochondrial myopathies, improved gait in my patients with neurodegenerative diseases, less pain in my patients with chronic pain syndromes, and even improved gut motility in my patients with gastroparesis and small intestinal bacterial overgrowth (SIBO). I have also seen improved joint function with local injections in my connective tissue disorder patients. And, importantly, I have seen improvement in fatigue in patients with chronic fatigue.

Exosomes are similarly effective against aging. Unlike stem cells, they are not autologous—they are not from the patient's own body—so you are getting someone else's DNA, but nevertheless they do many of the same things that stem cells do, albeit less sustained. They reduce inflammation, reduce pain, modulate the immune system, and enhance the regeneration of some tissue or the repair of some tissue. And they slow down aging.

Many patients, and people in general, are interested in products that are advertised as "anti-aging." Hand creams, face creams, masks, serums, and supplements. Sure, we all want to look younger, and where does our age show the most? Our skin. But in my opinion, the vast

---

1 It should be noted that use of stem cells is approved for certain devastating diseases. Stem cell transplants (after bone marrow ablation) are used for such diseases as adrenoleukodystrophy or primary progressive multiple sclerosis.

majority of these anti-aging products don't do anything. I'm a big advocate for collagen and feel it can do a lot of good for people with connective tissue disorders, and it's also good for the skin because skin is made of collagen. But even collagen supplements, like those powders that you put in your smoothie or protein shake—they are not very effective. However, I do recommend creams that contain GHK peptides. I usually provide it as an injectable for connective tissue disorders, but it also comes in creams, and GHK creams can be very effective in improving facial skin.

Other Regenerative Therapies

PROLOTHERAPY IS A DEXTROSE SOLUTION that is injected into a damaged joint to help rebuild collagen. It helps to promote healing by decreasing inflammation and pain and supporting the natural healing ability of the body, and it can be very effective for patients with connective tissue disorders. It can sometimes provoke a mast cell response, so it is important to manage and stabilize the mast cells. As an alternative therapy, it's not regulated by the FDA, but it has become fairly mainstream regardless, so be sure that you are getting treatment from a reputable provider. Ask your doctor or healthcare provider for guidance.

For damaged joints, damaged skin, or chronic muscle spasm, platelet-rich plasma (PRP) injections can be useful. To prepare a PRP injection, a healthcare technician will take your blood and spin it down so what is left is just plasma (no red blood cells) with platelets and growth factors. The platelets are concentrated up to eight times their normal number and mixed into a blood plasma liquid base and injected directly into the area of the injury. Once injected, the platelets repair the vessels that deliver the blood, and the growth factors spark a cascade of cellular repair and regeneration that can in time result in improved function and motion. Many patients can avoid, at the very least, years of increasing dosages of pain medications, and at the most, surgical reconstruction of their joints. PRP injections are fairly common now; you can ask your primary care doctor to refer you to a specialist, such as a physiatrist, pain or sports medicine specialist, or an orthopedist, who can administer the treatment.

A more expensive but also more effective treatment is plasmapheresis, which is basically a filtering of the patient's plasma. Your blood is taken and is separated into the plasma and cells. The cells are returned to you but the plasma is not—thereby removing autoantibodies, the antibodies that are attacking your body, and also removing inflammatory mediators, circulating viral RNA, and more. Then the filtered plasma is returned to the body. Plasmapheresis possibly filters out abnormal proteins for diseases like Alzheimer's and Parkinson's, and it is often used as a treatment for autoimmune diseases. It's been around for a hundred years, but it used to be intense and involve staying in the hospital or clinic. Now the technology has advanced to the point that it is much easier to do.

You can put a plasmapheresis machine in an office and do it on an outpatient basis. I'm bringing a machine into my office to treat my PEI patients because it's been shown to remove a lot of the mediators that are making them sick, such as circulating viral RNA and many of the mast cell mediators. Again, it's not cheap, and it is not going to be covered by insurance, but if you have access and can afford it, it's very effective. As a side note, plasmapheresis is another treatment that is great for combating aging, and it's very popular in the longevity movement. Some longevity fans get monthly plasmapheresis treatments. It's my hope that as the technology continues to advance, the cost will come down to where it's more accessible for everyone.

There are other regenerative therapies that you can do on your own, such as red-light therapy, a treatment that uses low-wavelength red light (which is different from infrared light) to stimulate the mitochondria in your cells. Mitochondria are commonly known as the energy powerhouse of your body because they are where energy production occurs, in the form of a molecule called adenosine triphosphate (ATP). With more energy, other cells can do their work more efficiently—work that includes reducing inflammation in cells, healing scars, producing more collagen, and increasing blood flow to tissues. You can buy a red light for use at home, with several high-quality options available online. I have one that I love, and so do several of my colleagues. If you do buy one, or if you consider using one at a beauty salon, spa, tanning salon, or wellness center, be sure to talk with your doctor or a healthcare provider about the best options. At-home lights may be less potent than medical-grade lights, but they can still be effective (and certainly more convenient). Red-light therapy is a great way to treat your symptoms.

If our bodies retain the ability to rebuild, we should allow that, for that holds power of not only no side effects but potential sustained response. But we do need to provide the right tools and the best internal environment to let it happen as optimally as possible, and regenerative therapies are those tools. They are safe and effective, and what is really exciting is that they are still developing and improving. We have not yet even scratched the surface. It's important, though, not to look at these as shortcuts or replacement for the lifestyle strategies discussed earlier in this book. There is no replacement for healthy living: smart diet, good sleep, activity and (if you are able) exercise, going outside and being exposed to light and abundant oxygen. With that foundation in place, or at least starting to be built up, you are already working on building up your stem cells, and from there other regenerative therapies can indeed be a way to make greater strides more quickly.

There are a lot of ideas in this chapter, and I know it can feel overwhelming to be faced with so many options. Peptide therapy can make some difference the fastest, but it is important to talk with your doctor before you get started.

It is important to decide what symptom or symptoms are most prominent in terms of interfering with your quality of life, your productivity, and your functionality, because sometimes, though not always, you can choose just where to begin on your own healing journey based on that symptom. Once you have been able to find consistency in your daily life with nutrition, movement, sleep, stress management, and more, then you can consider some of these other options that may require purchase of equipment or a little guidance from a knowledgeable healthcare provider.

Take-Home Guidelines

1. Our bodies have an amazing ability to heal themselves, and with regenerative therapies, we can expand that ability, resulting in remarkable healing of tissues damaged by chronic illness.
2. Some therapies involve taking materials from your own body and injecting them into affected areas, while others can use organic or other materials that you purchase.
3. Much of this you can do on your own, but you should talk to your doctor before starting.

10

Cleaning Up Your Environment

READ THIS CHAPTER TO FIND OUT . . .

- How toxicants creep into our environment in myriad ways
- How you can make lifestyle decisions to protect yourself

BY THE TIME I WAS in my fourth week of recovery from brain surgery, I had already made many changes to take control of my recovery. I had changed up my nutrition and was regularly juicing. I was going for daily walks. I was doing breathing exercises and practicing my meditation. I was taking some supplements to support my sleep and address neuroinflammation. And I had added hyperbaric oxygen and infrared sauna to my weekly recovery regimen.

Now that these fixes had begun to take effect and give me some energy and strength and hope, I was ready to turn to another kind of change—a change not to myself but to my home.

I was already choosing only organic foods when possible (though it was not always possible or even necessary). I took inventory of my cleaning products and my personal care products and began to research better, less toxic, more earth-sustaining products to use to clean my home and to take care of my skin, and then I slowly started to change what products I used. One big difference I noted early on was the less irritating odor of the products. I realized the previous products had been making me feel tired and irritable and causing headaches. But the new products had fewer toxic ingredients and more natural aromas, and I felt a lot better overall. My skin was less irritated and dry. I installed a filter in the sink in my kitchen to help remove impurities in the water. I had my home inspected for mold, and had my urine and blood tested for exposures and inflammatory markers, all of which, fortunately, were negative, and I placed air purifiers in most of the rooms in my house (this was years before Covid!). I made these changes, and I felt my recovery advance subtly. I felt good knowing that I was controlling the things I could control to reduce my exposures now and in the future. The best way to describe it is that I felt less contaminated.

The fact is, we can't control everything we are exposed to. Our environment keeps getting dirtier, and with each passing decade we are exposed to an increasing number of novel antigens that we are not prepared to deal with. Studies by the World Health Organization have shown that umbilical cord blood contains nearly 300 contaminants.[1] What this means is that we are already exposed from the day we are born. From there, the exposure only grows. Each day of our lives our bodies have to contend with the air we inhale, the food we eat, the water we drink, the pills we consume, the stuff we touch (including the potions we slather on our skin). And then we exhale, defecate and urinate, and bathe, therefore putting these same contaminants back into our environments—back into the air and wastewater systems— contributing to the continuous vicious cycle of exposure, and our bodies suffer under the weight.

The array of contaminants we're exposed to is wide ranging and includes pharmaceuticals, supplements, foods, personal care and beauty products, and cleaning products for our homes and offices, not to mention toxicants from industrial and agricultural practices. Regulations under international, federal, and state programs aim to prevent, control, and mitigate the presence and the effects of these pollutants. In the United States, the EPA is tasked with trying to study what levels humans can be exposed to without experiencing acute and potentially dangerous

---

1 "Body Burden: The Pollution in Newborns," Environmental Working Group, July 14, 2005, https://www.ewg.org/research/body-burden -pollution-newborns.

symptoms and increasing the risk for diseases such as cancer or respiratory ailments. Then the EPA must try to regulate the industries that make these noxious chemicals so that they don't spew more into our environment. It is a nearly impossible task especially as the regulatory authority of the EPA is being curtailed.[2]

Our level of exposure to these toxins may be small at any given time, but it is important to recognize that even at amounts so small they are measured in parts per billion, the cumulative exposure over decades of life contributes to, or at least puts us at risk for, chronic illness. These toxins weaken the immune system, weaken the connective tissue, and cause systemic and neural inflammation. It is amazing we stand at all.

We do not, at least individually, have much control over what pollution is emitted from regional and global industries, though we should remember that collectively we have a strong political voice. Regardless, we do have the means to reduce our exposure burden as a preventive measure and to help us recover from chronic illness. We can control the foods we eat, the beauty products we use, the cleaning agents we use, and, to some extent, the air we breathe and the medications and supplements we consume. Making smart decisions in these areas may not produce dramatic

---

2 Nina Totenberg, "Supreme Court Restricts the EPA's Authority to Mandate Carbon Emissions Reductions," NPR, updated June 30, 2022, https://www.npr.org/2022/06/30/1103595898/supreme-court-epa-climate-change.

changes right away, but over time they will help you (and your family or whoever else is exposed to the food and products you bring into your home) feel better and reduce your risk in the future.

Food

CONVENIENCE HAS BECOME A MARK of our society in many areas, and perhaps none more obviously than in the foods we eat. We demand convenience, and food corporations have delivered it, but the problem is that convenience leads to less healthy choices and hence more risk of inflammation and disease. There must be a balance we can achieve. Healthy food does not have to be inconvenient. Healthy food in the specific context of chronic illness of course refers to the nutritional value it holds but also to its being anti-inflammatory and free of environmental and industrial toxins, pesticides, herbicides, and other exposures. Bottom line: We choose the foods we eat, so we can make healthy choices.

As discussed in Chapter 5, I strongly recommend adopting a plant-based diet. The meat industry is trying to be friendlier to the earth and healthier for human bodies, but ultimately our bodies require a lot of energy to metabolize meats—energy that could be diverted to clearing the system of toxic metabolites. While fish is touted as a healthy food, the fat of fish bioaccumulates much of what is in our waters, including contaminants that have already been proven to be disruptive to the health and safety of nonhuman species that live in or by waterways, and ultimately lead to disease in these species. It is important to remember that waters are shared across the globe, so limit consumption of fish regardless of its body of water origin or its farming practice of origin.

It's also very important to buy organic, non-GMO foods. These foods are free of chemicals and preservatives that are dangerous to our biological systems and also devalue the nutritional component of our foods. Organic food is now more widely available and less expensive than ever before. It still does cost more than its conventional sister in many areas, though that is changing. Even so, I think it important to prioritize our health as best we can, so it is worth thinking about rebalancing how we spend our money so we can prioritize consuming more organic food. It is valid to consider the much greater cost—including the financial cost—to our health in the long term from many years of poor food choices.

It's not necessary to buy everything organic, but I definitely recommend going organic when purchasing foods from "The Dirty Dozen," a guide compiled annually by the Environmental Working Group. These twelve foods really should be eaten only in organic form because the conventionally raised form contains far too much in terms of chemicals, and the food itself is not covered in a skin that we peel or cut off. The Dirty Dozen are strawberries, spinach, dark leafy greens, cherries, blueberries, green beans, peaches, pears, nectarines, grapes, apples, and peppers. So even when we are trying to eat in an anti-inflammatory manner and are intentionally choosing these seemingly healthy fruits and vegetables, they are not clean if they're not organic, which means they can have adverse effects on our health. Synthetic chemicals and microbials and their toxins are more potent than the phytonutrients contained in any food that is grown from the earth. Organic produce and other food products have a significant advantage in this regard, so look for the U.S. Department of Agriculture (USDA) organic seal on foods you purchase. The USDA has strict standards for certifying a grower as organic, so if a food has that seal, it is at least 95 percent free of environmental exposures that serve to weaken our immune system and stoke systemic and neuroinflammatory fires. Foods labeled "100% Organic" are even better, as they contain only organic products.

Though it may be unpleasant to think about, we should consider what happens to our food after we eat it, too. Some of it enters the environment at some point, albeit in a different form and in different quantities. We excrete, urinate, exhale, and sweat metabolic waste by-products, and if our foods contain chemicals and synthetic derivatives, we are returning them to our water and soil systems, and thus they are being used to grow new produce that will now incorporate these contaminants, and the cycle starts anew. Regenerative farming techniques are being developed to nurture healthy soil and protect water resources, and I am proud to be part of the Kiss the Ground movement, but the more we consume foods laden with contaminants and toxicants, the more of an uphill battle it will be.

Personal Care Products

WE SLATHER CREAMS, LOTIONS, OILS, and oint-ments on our face and body. We wash our hair, paint our nails, apply makeup, and brush our teeth. The products we use to do all this make it back to the environment when we bathe, circling the drain before making their way into the pipelines that take them back into the environment. And just like the trash that is hauled away from our homes, the residue from these personal care products do not vanish and are not gone. They do not dissipate or evaporate, though some condense and enter the air as particles. They make their way through pipes and into wastewater that then makes its way to treatment plants for processing, only to return to our drinking water. It is not of little importance to note that most water treatment facilities do not contain technology that can remove these toxic compounds.

We can be very susceptible to marketing schemes and advertisements that promise youthful-looking skin, prevention of the telltale signs of aging, and healthy hair and nails. Often our vanity clouds our thinking about what we are doing to the environment with these products, to say nothing of what we're doing to our bodies. Fortunately, there has been an exponential increase in the past decade of natural and organic personal care and beauty products available to us. These products are manufactured by companies that are dedicated to reducing toxic exposure to the planet and to humans, and so they contain only ingredients that are less toxic and polluting to our bodies or the world around us. They also use recycled and biodegradable packaging.

But it's important to be careful about the products you choose. The word "natural" implies ingredients that are derived from nature and not created in a lab, but the FDA does not regulate that term, so in truth, any company can label any product as "natural." It's also true that sometimes natural ingredients are unsafe for us, particularly if they contain toxic heavy metals or cause an allergic reaction. The term "organic" can be tricky, too. As with foods, it is regulated by the USDA, but look for the "USDA Organic" seal. A product can say "organic" without actually being approved by the USDA, so make sure it has that seal. Even terms like "hypoallergenic" and "dermatologist tested" can, unfortunately, be basically meaningless. To help consumers make the best decisions when buying personal products, the Mayo Clinic has developed a free app called SkinSafe. As they say, Mayo Clinic experts have "done all the label reading for you," so you can simply scan barcodes when shopping and get a safety rating as well as an analysis of ingredients that can provide some peace of mind.

Electronic Devices

Our personal electronic products are almost like an extension of ourselves. We rarely leave home without our phones, and our tablets and computers are basically always on. There is not yet clear evidence of the damage that electromagnetic radiation fields can induce, but that does not mean that the radiation our devices emit is not potentially damaging. Limiting the use of screens will reduce your exposure and have the added benefits of improved sleep, improved mental health, and more free time to dedicate to your health. In addition to limiting screen time during the day, turn off phones, tablets, and WiFi at night to reduce radiation exposure. Limit your conversations with a handheld cell phone held to your ear to three minutes.

Cleaning Products

WE ALL LIKE A CLEAN home, a clean car, a clean office, and clean clothes. But the products we use to achieve that level of cleanliness hold the same risk as personal care and beauty products. An important distinction is that they are not intended to be applied directly to the human body in any way, but that does not make them less dangerous. In fact, because they are not intended for human use, the standards by which they are regulated are lower and less rigid, so these products are usually more toxic than personal care and beauty products. Commercial cleaning products that come in sprays are not only applied to the countertops from which we prepare and eat food or other applications, but they enter the air via aerosol and nozzle sprays. We easily inhale these particles and noxious fumes, and they also settle on our skin—an important organ that is meant to serve as a barrier to protect our internal environment, but one that is easily breached. This is especially concerning in the context of chronic inflammatory illness with widespread involvement of connective tissue, including the collagen layers of our skin.

Similar to personal care and beauty products, there are many sustainable and "green" cleaning products available. When they were first on the market more than a decade ago, they were very expensive, and many people simply could not afford to purchase them. But as time has gone on and interest in living in a more sustainable fashion has increased, formulations have improved, and these products have become less expensive. More products are designed to contain more water-soluble ingredients and fewer synthetic chemicals that can be damaging to the environment and to species that rely on clean water and healthy soil for their lives, as well as ingredients that can be very inflammatory to human bodies.

Again, you need to be wary about labeling and product claims. The terms "green," "eco-friendly," "nontoxic," and "sustainable" are not regulated and therefore are essentially meaningless. As with food, the USDA will apply its "Certified Organic" seal to products that meet its standards for organic products, but again, the word "organic" on a product is not regulated and therefore not helpful without that seal. As with food, you can't trust the word "natural," either, but look for the USDA's "Certified Biobased" seal, which will include a number that tells you the exact percentage of the product that is biobased. There is also a very helpful non-government organization: A nonprofit called the ToxicFree Foundation maintains a free database of "green light ingredients," which are guaranteed to be free of harmful chemicals, and "red light ingredients," which do contain unsafe chemicals, so you can look up the stuff that's in the products you own or are considering buying.

Sporadic and occasional use of personal care and cleaning products probably will not do much harm, and I hate to be an alarmist or run around like Chicken Little, but most of these products we don't use sporadically. We don't wash our face every now and then, we do it every day. The same goes for applying lotion and cleaning our space and belongings. It is in the context of the overall exposure burden that we look for ways we can perhaps control, even if minimally, the dangers that lurk.

Medications

MOST PATIENTS WITH CHRONIC ILLNESS take an average of five medications, often prescribed by more than one doctor. Many symptoms of chronic illness can be relieved with pharmacological options, and each doctor a patient sees may offer a different, new, or alternative medication plan. Does this sound familiar? You may go through a series of medication trials and continue some medications and discontinue others, and after a few years you have accumulated multiple vials of drugs that are stockpiled in the cabinet. I have had patients on ten to fifteen medications.

"Polypharmacy," a term loosely defined as when one person is actively taking more than five medications, is known to be a risk factor for many symptoms, so reducing your pharmacological intake can be an important piece of your overall care plan on its own. I ask patients to write a spreadsheet that lists their medications, dosing, and frequency of administration, and then add who prescribed each one, when, and why. Learning the indication for each prescription is important, because then we can discuss in depth the symptom each medication is intended to treat and what has been its effect since the patient started on the medication. Then we compare each medication with the other medications on the list to see where there is overlap in terms of what they are supposed to do. I have often been able to streamline a patient's cocktail of medications so that they are taking fewer, and taking ones that seem to be having a positive effect on their disease.

The reason this matters is that medications do come with the risk, albeit rare, of toxicity, especially for chronic illness patients whose immune system is on high alert. The toxicity can result from the biologically active formula in medications, one of the many excipients that are added to help preserve or stabilize the formulation, or a combination of the two, especially when one is taking multiple medications. Adverse reactions and sensitivity to drugs may be triggered by the compound itself or its excipients. In fact, many patients with mast cell activation disorders are not able to tolerate many medications at all unless they are compounded, meaning the biologically active formula is capsulized or packaged in some form without excipients. Not all medications are amenable to this process, but most are, and I recommend getting your medications compounded if you can.

The other source of exposure is how we dispose of the medications that end up stockpiled and expired in our medicine cabinets. We flush them down the toilet or spill them into the sink. The Office of National Drug Control Policy of the White House released guidelines on how to dispose of drugs, with a focus on narcotics so they were not available for theft, by pulverizing them and mixing them with coffee grounds, putting them in a box, wrapping them in tape, and disposing of them in the garbage. I was also instrumental during my dissertation days helping various cities in the country set up "drug take-back" days, which are days when the public could return their unused medications to their pharmacies. These days, different municipalities have changed to include other drop-off locations, including police stations and city waste locations.

While these are still real options for disposal, most of us do not have the time or the energy to follow through with these methods, which leaves our waterways as the most convenient method of disposal. Even disposing of the unused medication in the garbage means they end up in landfills and leach into the underground water and eventually the community water systems. This contributes to the exposure burden for all, makes us sick, and makes the sick even sicker. Studies have shown that species that live in or by the water have suffered from the pharmaceutical residues identified in these waterways. These species have aberrations of sex differentiations, congenital abnormalities, and other physiological changes that affect their feeding, migration, and mating habits.

Therefore, minimal prescribing of the lowest effective dose is an important tactic that you and your doctor can take. Especially for the concern of hypersensitivity in patients with chronic illness, doctors should start with a low dose. For your part as the patient, communicate often regarding tolerance and response. Starting with lower doses may mean that it takes longer to find that a medication does indeed provide improvement, but that process helps you lower your exposure to drug compounds and excipients as well as your secondhand exposure via the environment, because you will have less to dispose of and excrete. It also helps to protect the environment.

Obviously, I absolutely do not recommend that you stop taking any medication without consulting with a doctor first, but you can jump-start that conversation with your doctor by creating your own spreadsheet or handwritten list of your medications and bringing it in to them. Make a grid or spreadsheet with four columns. Label the first column "Medication," and fill that column with the name of each of the medications you are taking. The second column is "Dose," where you fill in the dosage for the medication in each row, and the third is "Frequency," or how many times a day you take it. Label the fourth column "Purpose," and for each medication write down why you are taking that particular medication. (This one sometimes stumps my patients who have been taking a lot of medication for a long time.)

When You Talk to Your Doctor About . . . Your Medication List

Once you have compiled your list of medications and filled in all the other columns of information for each one, give each drug some thought. If it's intended to reduce pain, for example, try to be objective with yourself about whether it has been effective at all. How much change, if any, have you noticed since you started on that medication? Also, does it produce any side effects? Take note of those, too. When you bring your list to your doctor, have notes prepared regarding your experience as well as any questions or concerns you have regarding each medication, with the intent of learning more about the drugs that have been prescribed to you. You hold autonomy, and you should have informed consent for all that is suggested, recommended, and prescribed.

Treat this as a learning mission at first. One thing you're learning is the landscape of your pharmacological intake, which can often be an eye-opening experience on its own. At the same time, your doctor may not be fully aware of how many different medications and/or supplements you are taking, especially if you see multiple doctors, or how their usage may be overlapping or competing with one another, so it might be a learning experience for them, too. Be clear that you are interested in reducing the number of medications you take if that is safe and will not slow your recovery. And if you and your doctor are in agreement with discontinuing one or more of your medications, be sure you understand what the recommended weaning schedule is so you do it in a safe manner with as few risks as possible.

Supplements

PATIENTS OFTEN FIND THE LANDSCAPE of supplements to be vast and confusing, unhelpful at best and harmful at worst. Broadly speaking, most supplements are a waste of money, though I do have a few that I recommend.

One of the biggest problems, as we have discussed, is that supplements, probably more than most medications, are filled with excipients. This is because they must have a long shelf life and so they must be preserved as they sit on the shelves of stores and warehouses. They are also not regulated, so the amount of the actual compound you are buying—the vitamin, mineral, nutrient—is typically very small in the product, partly because larger amounts may pose a potential health risk to certain subsets of the population (which may include those with chronic illness). In fact, some studies have shown that the concentration of the targeted compound is very small in some brands, if it even exists at all.[3] So when consuming supplements, we are mainly consuming the excipients. Compounding supplements, which I discussed in Chapter 5 and which can be done in some circumstances, can be very expensive and likely not worth the cost unless there is a particular compound a patient is truly in need of and that is known to be effective for a particular symptom. Especially when considering the need for long-term use, your money is probably better spent getting that nutrient from an actual food source, which is more effective anyway. (See pages 133–135 for guidelines on juicing for specific nutrients.)

Another problem is that patients are often counseled to try multiple supplements by multiple doctors, even more so than medications. Sometimes there's a conflict of interest when doctors sell the supplements in their practices and are pushing them to make money, and many have even developed a line of privately labeled supplements. Things get even more messy because anyone can recommend or sell supplements since they do not require a prescription. Supplements tend to be recommended by almost anyone a patient sees, including acupuncturists, massage therapists, chiropractors, physical therapists and naturopathic doctors, resulting in frequent and commonly contradictory

---

3 Giovanna Esposito et al., "Disclosing Frauds in Herbal Food Supplements Labeling: A Simple LC-MS/MS Approach to Detect Alkaloids and Biogenic Amines," *Journal of Food Protection* 86, no. 10 (October 2023): https://doi.org/10.1016/j.jfp.2023.100152.

recommendations of supplements. It can be confusing and frustrating when you are being told you should take this or take that by so many voices, and many of my patients end up with twenty to thirty bottles or vials of supplements in their regimen. To sort things out if you are taking a lot of supplements, you may want to write up a spreadsheet in the same fashion as you did for prescribed medications. It can be harder to interpret exactly what supplement is having what effect because the bioavailability—meaning how much is made available to the body—of the desired compound is not readily known, nor is the extent of your compliance in taking the supplement—which can be spotty—so it may not be worth your time to try to sort it all out. But at least it can give you and your doctors a snapshot of all that you are taking, which can be a valuable learning experience in itself.

Finally, just as with medications, all the compounds and excipients that come in supplements have an ultimate destination—whether we consume or dispose of them—that leads to either direct or indirect exposure to our bodies and our environmental surroundings. Our goal must be to reduce the burden on our bodies by minimizing supplemental use to what is clearly beneficial and has sound theoretical basis for continued use.

The first rule of thumb for reducing supplement usage is to only use supplements to target a specific symptom and not for overall well-being. I generally recommend avoiding multivitamins because most of what is in them is not

bioavailable, and honestly, if you eat even a minimal variety of foods you will get the vitamins you need. Next,
be precise and deliberate about the supplements you use.
When initiating treatment, use them only as support for
medications and other treatments—supplements alone
are not potent enough to improve suffering. They do not
work fast, and they need to be taken in a very strict and
rigid manner without missing many doses. After that, they
can certainly be used for maintenance and possible prevention once symptoms are improving, but again, be sure
you are targeting specific symptoms and being conservative
in choosing what to take. Refer to Chapter 5 for a deeper
discussion of which supplements you should consider and
which you should avoid, but suffice it to say that I strongly
recommend tincture, liquid, or powered formulations rather
than capsulized because they are more effective and contain
fewer excipients.

Whatever supplements you do take, it is worth your
time to find brands that are of high quality. Of course,
supplements are unregulated, so there is no stamp or
certificate that reliably indicates quality, making this a
tricky business to figure out. Your doctor may be able to
help guide you. Often, doctors sell or recommend certain
brands because they trust them but, as I have said, other
times doctors are simply selling brands to make money.
It's helpful if you have a strong therapeutic relationship
with your doctor and you trust them. Beyond that, I have
vetted many brands and have found three that I'm satisfied

with—or I should say *was* satisfied with when I did that research, which was in 2016, since I do not have the time to keep up with changes in any companies or to monitor new companies that come on the scene. Based on my vetting at that time, the brands I most trust are Thorne, Pure Encapsulations, and Vital Nutrients. Recently, because of my work with other clinicians and scientists, I also trust supplements offered by neuroneeds.com and algonot.com.

Air and Water

THE AIR WE BREATHE IS the only air we have, and it puts us at risk for myriad exposures. Droplets and aerosols carry infectious organisms and other toxic particles. Wildfires fill our air with smoke even in areas that are remote from the fire itself. Weather patterns affected by climate change and industry and agriculture have greatly worsened the quality of our air in general. While these are all sad signs of the times, we are not powerless to do anything. Here are a few guidelines and suggestions:

- To start, it is imperative to have air filters and purifiers in our homes, preferably in each room we spend a lot of time in such as living rooms, bedrooms, and offices. Fortunately, the technology of standalone air purifiers has greatly improved in recent years, making them more affordable and more effective.

- This will come as a bummer to many, but we all should continue to wear masks when we go out in public where there will be people in close proximity to us and where we are in enclosed or partially enclosed places, not only because SARS-CoV-2 is still a threat, but because so are other viruses and toxins in the air. I cannot imagine a future where I do not wear a mask in crowded places such as planes and airports.
- Deep breathing exercises can aid the exchange and removal process to further clean out the airways of our lungs.
- Get outdoors and exercise or move. Despite the concerns about particulate matter in the air, studies have proven that exposure to nature (as opposed to city and urban environments) allows for improved detoxification as a result of the symbiotic relationship humans have with flora and fauna.
- We could all benefit from occasional oxygen therapy.

Similarly, the water we drink is limited to what is available to us in our individual municipality. Not only are we exposed to toxicants in our drinking water (including many pharmaceutical residues), but we are also adding to them through the things we as humans do to the environment. To avoid further polluting and destroying the environment, use reusable water bottles and avoid disposable plastic water bottles. To better protect yourself from the many toxicants in water, purchase a filtering system for your home sink, or at least get a filtered pitcher like a Brita to keep in your refrigerator or use filters for the dispensers that are fitted for the doors of your refrigerator. Water treatment plants have come a long way and do an impressive job cleaning our water, and the water in most cities is pretty good. But even our best technology can't remove everything, and sometimes contaminants are picked up after water leaves the plant by way of what it's exposed to in the pipes. Personal water filters are not perfect, either, but they provide an additional layer of protection.

In the end, that is all we can do with any of these potential toxins and toxicants—limit our exposure. It can be frustrating and even infuriating to realize that we cannot, in this modern world, eliminate all exposures and live in a clean, or mostly clean, environment, but that is no reason to throw our hands up and give in. Let's not allow perfect to be the enemy of the good. As with so many of the changes and treatments I'm suggesting in this book, we do have the power to make things better, and better is, well, better. Clean living is possible, just as recovery is possible, even if we have to take baby steps at times.

Take-Home Guidelines

1. Adopt a plant-based diet and purchase organic, non-GMO foods when possible and when necessary (like when buying "The Dirty Dozen").
2. Use only organic and clean personal products and cleaning products.

3. Consult with your doctor to get a handle on the medications and supplements you are taking and strive to reduce them. Polypharmacy is real and can cause problems, and use of multiple supplements is an expensive and not necessarily therapeutic habit.

4. Buy and use air filters and water filters.

PART III

Determination and Diligence

11

The Hero of Your Story

OVER A RECENT HOLIDAY WEEKEND, I visited my daughter in Philadelphia. I stayed in a hotel near her apartment, but for three days I spent nearly every waking hour with her, sinking into her life in a way I had not been able to do since she left home two years ago—or, honestly, since she was much younger. I'm deeply proud of her, and I'm so happy that she seems to be doing well, but sometimes I walk past her bedroom at home and suddenly miss her so much that I have to sit down. So being with her in her world, meeting her friends, cooking with her, talking with her about her classes, watching a movie together while snuggling on her couch, all of this was a lovely salve for the soul.

On Sunday I left Philadelphia for New York, where I worked for a week at Mount Sinai Hospital. I could have done these two trips separately, but I wanted to combine them into one, which seemed more efficient even though I knew it would be exhausting. My work in New York was intense and consuming, and again I lived out of a hotel, and when I finally flew home after being away for ten days, I was indeed emotionally and physically exhausted. Not only that, but I had also completely fallen out of my usual health regimen while I was gone. I hadn't been able to eat the foods I wanted to eat. I could not exercise on a regular basis in the ways that I wanted to exercise, and I did not sleep well because I never sleep well in hotels. Everything I do and have done since my surgery to keep myself feeling good and functional was totally out of whack. And the day after I got home, I woke up and felt the worst I had felt in probably a year. I mean I felt like shit. I had a horrible headache, I was nauseated and dizzy, and I could barely get out of bed. I thought I might have caught Covid on the trip, but the test was negative. It was not Covid or the flu, it was just stress and travel and—most important—not doing the things I do to keep myself well.

I got up and started my routine. I went outside to get some sun. I made my green juice and drank it. I did my exercises, and I got back onto my schedule. I took care of myself, and you know what? The next day I woke up and felt great.

I am the first to admit that this isn't easy. Chronic complex illness is scary and mysterious. Many of the treatments are arduous. They take a lot of work and a lot of tenacity, and it's easy to make a mistake. Maybe one night you stay up too late with friends, you eat pizza and drink beer, and the next day you feel terrible. It's harder to wake up on time, harder to exercise, and you're craving less-than-healthy comfort food all day, and all that makes it hard to get back to doing those things that help you feel good. And listen, if having a couple beers is how you have fun with friends, you deserve to do that now and then. I am not here judging you one bit. Maybe you like to treat yourself to dessert once in a while, or you skip your work-out sometimes. It's okay. I'm not beating myself up over my double-down trip to the East Coast. Life gets in the way sometimes, and you can't eat or sleep or work out the way you need to. It's okay.

My point is that you are in charge. If your journey toward recovery were a road trip, you would be the driver. If it were a movie, you would be the hero. Which means the responsibility for facing the villain—your illness—lies with you. More important, the *power* lies with you. As I have said a few times in this book, every day presents a new opportunity to make a good choice. If you don't have the energy or resources to make a big decision, make a smaller one. You don't have to go vegan overnight. But you can make some changes. Take a swing at that villain. As you start to feel better, take more. Remember that you don't have to be perfect. All you have to do is your best. Do what you can, and be diligent, and with each decision you make, pay attention to how your body feels.

This also applies to treatments you undergo with the help of your doctor. You will probably not find the right medications after one visit to the clinic. Your pharmacological needs will probably change over time, too. Again, the key is to be diligent and pay attention to how your body feels. And communicate with your doctor.

Seek a Strong Therapeutic Relationship

I HAVE MENTIONED THE DOCTOR-PATIENT relationship a few times. It is so important to build this relationship up. When I see a patient, as I have said, I spend a lot of time with them to figure out exactly how to help them. I do an extensive workup to try to find where I can intervene for this particular patient. What can we do that will be the most use, that will give us the most bang for the buck? Today I saw three patients who all have the same post-exposure chronic illness, but they're all on different plans. I check in with each of them regularly to see how their plan is working, how they are feeling, and we change path when it appears that we need to change path. One of them has a copper deficiency, and I'm trying to figure out what that might mean and what I can do about it. The reason I do this is because there is no blueprint for treating chronic complex illness, even when people have the same exact illness. Every body reacts in its own way.

When you have a strong relationship with your doctor, they are more likely to dive deep with you in this way to figure out your complex chronic illness. There's a greater chance the doctor will look carefully at the medications you are taking and listen to what you say about how they make you feel, and they may say back to you, for example, "Hey, this medication is working well for you and it also helps with so and so, let's think about that. Let's connect these two things you're feeling and see if we can get some traction this other way." Your doctor may then consider options with a similar way of working, or additional options that add to the initial treatment, or even non-medication therapies that can support or enhance what has already been effective. For example, a patient with severe brain fog due to neuroinflammation had great relief with medications that thinned the blood and protected the lining of the vessel wall. To further enhance response, we started nitric oxide lozenges, which help open up vessels to further improve blood flow, and palmitoylethanolamide to hasten the reduction of inflammation, and omega-3 oil to support blood thinning and vessel lining protection. The road for this patient was long, and we had tried multiple medications until we found one and then two that offered clinical benefit—which happened to be an immunotherapy drug. Because we had developed a relationship of communication and trust, we were able to connect on a level that was ultimately therapeutic. I understood her symptoms more and more over the visits, and our discussions grew deeper, and she understood my thought process and goals for her from those same discussions.

Nurturing that kind of relationship can take time, dedication, understanding, care, and patience. That sounds like a tall order, I know, and often you are just not feeling well enough to even consider investing any of your short supply of energy into building a therapeutic connection with your doctor, who by cultural and historical expectation is already supposed to be dedicated to helping you (ideally this would always be the case, and it still often is). But doctors are overworked and overburdened. And while that is not your fault or your problem, the doctor–patient relationship does take a little more work and, dare I say, humanity these days.

Remember, too, that this is a two-way relationship, and just like any other relationship, both people need to contribute. If your doctor is not willing to entertain your concerns and your fears and take you seriously, maybe that's not your doctor. That does not mean you burn through doctors at the first hint of a slight. This happens to be a therapeutic relationship, where one of you is labeled doctor and one is labeled patient, but you're still just humans, and sometimes people are in a bad mood, and sometimes they have a personality or life experience that leads them to interpret things a certain way or receive things in a certain way, or they react to things a certain way, and you may have to learn about each other as you go. You learn how best to approach a topic with an individual. That's what I have done with my patients and even with my doctors, because there is no other choice. I have several doctors on my team, and I talk to them differently just based on what I have learned about their personalities. And that's not a bad thing. We are not robots; we are not all the same. We are all humans.

In the end, though, the unfortunate truth is that many

doctors are not willing or, more likely, able to do the hard work that it takes to truly address your chronic illness. It takes a lot of time and many visits, and they often do not have the support and resources they would need to do the job for you well. All you can really do is give your doctor the information about your symptoms, your concerns, and your fears and hope they will be able to find a way to offer some minimal guidance—even if at first it does not seem like they are going to work out. Remembering that they are human, you can say, "Well, that first appointment was not all that great. But maybe I'll give them a second chance and have a plan for approaching them differently next time." Or maybe the next time they will be prepared with recommendations that can actually help get you on your way.

And if after that second visit you still don't feel like your doctor is listening to you and seeing you, then walk away. It is okay. There are other doctors, and not every patient and doctor are a good fit.

Gather Support

I HOPE YOU ARE LUCKY enough (or persistent enough) to find a doctor who will go on this journey with you. I hope, too, that you have people in your private life who support you in the many ways you need it. It does not have to be a spouse or partner, though it is obviously wonderful if you do have a supportive partner. It could be parents or other family or close friends. It could be someone unexpected, perhaps someone who has been through a similar experience and wants to offer their wisdom and help. With any luck, it is several of these people. As a doctor, I know for a fact that patients do better with a good support system. When you have someone on your side who is supportive—not just emotionally but also physically in the moment, making meals and doing laundry and getting you to the clinic and so on—you have a better chance at recovery. I see it every day, because many of my patients bring their person into the office, and I get to hear from them, too, and see that relationship and what kind of help the patient is getting.

I also know this from my time as a patient. During those weeks when I was recovering from surgery, I took great strength from my husband's optimism and steadfastness and his literally doing everything I needed. I was buoyed by my daughter's love and her regular company in my bedroom, especially when she made just the right wisecrack to snap me out of a bout of self-pity and gloom. (Even though my skull hurt like hell when I laughed.) And when I was despairing because I couldn't eat because every move of my jaw led to intense, searing pain, and I was beginning to imagine a tragicomic scene in which I starved to death in a house full of food, my friend Deirdre came over and began juicing meals for me. She bought me my first juicer and shared with me her favorite recipes, and before long I was gaining strength. She also helped me to wash my greasy, dried blood–filled hair in the sink while my staples were still in, which helped me start to feel like a human again.

I could have made it through without all that support, but I shudder to think what it would have been like. Besides being lonelier, it would have been a lot harder in every way, and I have no doubt it would have been slower.

If you don't have the support you need, please ask for it. It helps to be specific. Instead of "I could use your help," try "Could you get me a protein smoothie?" Or "I need a ride to the doctor on Tuesday, can you help me out?" Many people want to help, but most of the time they don't know what you need. Many will reflexively bring food, and that can be helpful, but it may be that what you really need is someone to pick up your prescription. Or walk with you around the block, supporting you if you falter. Or just sit and watch TV with you one night. Whatever it is, ask for it. You will probably find that your journey leads not only to recovery but also to more substantial relationships.

Again, though, no matter who is in your support system and who your doctor is, remember that you are the hero of your story. That may seem like a lonely position to be in, and it may feel overwhelming. Some of the things I have talked about in this book may seem dark. The mystery and the lack of a clear road map for what you have been going through and what you can expect can be discouraging. I understand that all too well. But this does not have to feel hopeless. Rather, I think it is the single biggest source of hope. You can be the one to make changes. You can be the one to sleuth out what is helping and what is hurting. All you have to do is do. To me, that is empowering. I look at the stories of so many of my patients, and I see heroes. I picture you reading this, taking control of your story, and I see the same thing.

A Vision of the Future

WILL YOU EVER BE "NORMAL" again?

It's a question I hear often from patients, and unfortunately—if by "normal" you mean a full return to the person you were before this chronic illness, with 100 percent of the same physical condition and abilities—I can't promise that you will. The fact is that your physiology has changed, and it will remain changed forevermore. However, if you care for yourself, if you remain diligent in the ways we have discussed, and if you attend to your body and listen to the signals it sends you, not only when you feel lousy but every day, even when you feel great, then you have a great chance of being well. Very well, even. Certainly, you will be able to engage in work and family opportunities, you will be able to enjoy a social life. And I think that's pretty good, and that's worth fighting for, because tomorrow is not promised to any of us. You will always have to make greater efforts than you did before, greater than most people have to make, but hey—the world is trying to kill all of us. We are here to fight back and hopefully create a better world in doing so. But the experience of chronic illness and how it changes your life can have lasting effects—even once you have improved. There is a level of post-traumatic stress from the experience itself and the loss of quality life time that cannot be ignored, and I also help patients deal with those symptoms, too, when the time comes.

It's worth pointing out that medicine is improving all the time. Researchers are researching, technology is advancing, and critically, more and more doctors are opening up to the mysteries and taking the time to truly understand their patients' symptoms and reactions. There is momentum for sure, and I want us all to take advantage of it. Ten years ago, there was no such thing as commercially available peptide therapy. Incredible tools and modalities such as the Gyrotonic system and infrared saunas have grown from embryonic ideas to promising breakthroughs to proven therapies in a few short years, and they are becoming more common everywhere. These are just a few examples. There may be no blueprint, but we are learning more every day. The future looks better all the time.

My ten-day trip to Philadelphia and New York did set me back for a day, but the truth is that I never could have gone on that trip in the first place if not for my steadfast work in attending to my health. My doctors did not expect me to make it this far, but my story has not been a fluke. It will end eventually, of course. But I have a lot more to do before then, and I intend to keep being the hero of that story. You can do the same thing. You have that power.

How to Treat Common Post-Exposure Illness Symptoms Non-Pharmacologically

PLEASE FIRST SEE YOUR DOCTOR to rule out underlying conditions that may cause any of these symptoms. Also note the following may help minimize the symptom but will likely not result in sustained resolution.

NAUSEA

- Ginger tea, juice (juice it yourself!), candy, and ale
- Compression wristbands
- Peppermint tea
- Licorice tincture
- Marshmallow tincture
- Tonic water

- IV hydration with Ringer's lactate
- Acupressure
- Biofeedback
- TMS
- Deep breathing
- Lying flat on floor, knees bent, mild pressure with hands over belly button
- Walking in nature
- Ice on temples (cold cap), chest
- Cranial sacral therapy

DIZZINESS

- Deep breathing
- Hydration with electrolytes
- Slow movements as you change position
- Feet flat on floor for five minutes when going from sitting to standing
- Yoga: child's pose
- Cold shower
- Acupressure at region between eyes above nose (glabella)
- Acupressure above lip and below nose (philtrum)
- Lying flat on floor, knees bent, arms outstretched with palms pushing down into the floor

ABDOMINAL PAIN

- Walking
- Peppermint tea
- Ginger tea
- Castor oil packs
- Abdominal massage
- Cold packs on stomach while lying on your back
- Stretch with arms high to lengthen contents of abdominal cavity (can be standing or lying on your back)
- Yoga: happy baby pose

HEADACHE

- Chew on rosemary herb
- Rosemary tea
- Cold cap
- Cold shower with cold water directed at face, throat, chest
- Cold compress on throat and chest
- Acupressure at supraorbital notch on both sides (the area directly under the eyebrows and closest to the nose)
- Acupressure above the lips under the nose (philtrum)
- Manual traction to lift head up off neck (be mindful of placement of fingers, amount of traction, and anatomical plane of traction)
- Small amount of carbohydrates

- Caffeine
- Salt water
- Sleep

BODY PAIN

- Compression gear
- Massage
- Infrared sauna
- Lidocaine patches (4 percent lidocaine patches are available over the counter)
- Physical therapy
- Hemp seed oil capsules
- CBD cream
- PEMF devices

BRAIN FOG

- Berberine
- Boswellia
- Infrared sauna
- Movement, stretching, exercise
- Deep breathing
- Walking outdoors
- Caffeine

- Blood flow restriction and release with movement
- HBOT

ABNORMAL MOVEMENTS (TWITCH, JERK-LIKE, TIC-LIKE, POSTURING)

- Change position (a position that can be helpful is a fetal position)
- Warm compress
- Compression gear
- Dopamine and phosphatidylserine foods—bananas, blueberries, white beans, soybeans
- Mucuna pruriens
- Oil of oregano
- Arnica cream massage
- Stretching exercises
- Vagal nerve stimulator
- Lidocaine patches (4 percent lidocaine patches are available over the counter)

Acknowledgments

I hold incredible gratitude for Jenara Nerenberg, my literary agent, who reached out to me in November 2021, convinced me I had a book to write, and was the best guide and support and cheerleader I could have asked for. Jenara instilled confidence I did not have in my ability to actually do this, helped me write the proposal, and led me to Eileen Rothschild and Char Dreyer and all those at St. Martin's Press who also believed in me and have been nothing short of incredible during this process that I was once so unfamiliar with. I was guided by each at every step of the way. I also need to thank Eric Braun for helping me with editing and streamlining my runaway thoughts and rambling ideas and concepts, which was no small task. His patience and insight into what I was trying to communicate was time-saving but also sanity saving.

ABOUT THE AUTHOR

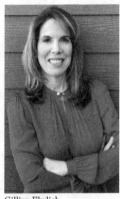

Gillian Ehrlich

DR. ILENE RUHOY is a neurologist and environmental toxicologist who specializes in chronic and complex illness. She graduated from the University of Pittsburgh School of Medicine, completed her residency in neurology at the University of Washington, and earned a PhD in environmental toxicology at the University of Nevada. In addition to her private practice in Seattle, Dr. Ruhoy serves as a medical director, coeditor, and speaker on the role of connective tissue in neurological disease.